HEART RENDING

HEART MENDING

Saved By Medical Science

Healed By Ancient Wisdom

D1127894

OTHER BOOKS BY MARYLOU KELLY STREZNEWSKI

Poetry

Rag Time
2002 J.G. Whitthorne Press

Woman Words
2003 J. G. Whitthorne Press

Dying with Robert Mitchum
2015 Aldrich Press

Non-Fiction

Gifted Grownups:
The Mixed Blessing of Extraordinary Potential
1999 John Wiley & Sons

For more about these books, visit:

http://streznewskiwrites.com

HEART RENDING

HEART MENDING

Saved By Medical Science
Healed By Ancient Wisdom

MARYLOU KELLY STREZNEWSKI, M. Ed.

For Glenda,
Best wishes,
M.K. Streznewski
March, 2017

J. G. WHITTHORNE PRESS

HEART RENDING

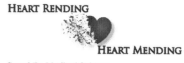

HEART MENDING

Saved By Medical Science
Healed By Ancient Wisdom

For more information visit: www.streznewskiwrites.com

Cover image: istockphoto.com/kirstypargeter
Cover and book design by Marie@DCS Book Designs

Printing History: First Printing 2015

Published by Create Space (a division of Amazon) for
J.G. Whitthorne Press
22 Brook Drive,
Furlong, PA 18925-1037

PRINTED IN THE UNITED STATES OF AMERICA
10 9 8 7 6 5 4 3 2 1

DEDICATION

To Dr. James McClurkin,
who saved me,

To Dr. Renee Sangrigoli,
who puts up with me,

To my husband Tom,
who stands by me,

And to the 64% who
can no longer speak,
especially Liz and Jan.

ACKNOWLEDGEMENTS

My greatest thanks go out to Marie Duess, a great friend who shepherded me through the labyrinth of preparing this book for publication, to Dr. Lana Liberto, who read the manuscript and offered helpful criticism, and to Karen Leahy who edited the manuscript. My sister-writers in the International Women's Writing Guild offered loving scoldings which kept me writing. The members of my Bucks County writing community encouraged me to include my poetry as part of the book, and were understanding when I wasn't around for class. My husband Tom was always available to solve my computer problems and provide the essential emotional support. Special thanks go to Dr. Mimi Guarneri and her belief that this book could save lives. May it be so.

TABLE OF CONTENTS

FOREWORD

There is an old saying: When the student is ready, the teacher will appear. I found this to be true in 1996, when my typical day of surgically opening blocked coronary arteries with small metal stents was interrupted by Dr. Dean Ornish, who asked me to lead a study to research the effectiveness of integrative medicine on critically ill heart patients. I had been placing stents in patients for years–that was how I treated patients with blocked arteries. I had never considered teaching them to eat a vegetarian diet, practice yoga, or meditate. I had never even tried yoga. But when Dean appeared outside of my lab, I knew I was ready to try a new approach.

Not only did I conduct the research, I participated in every step alongside my patients. We practiced yoga, meditated, and shared our experiences in support groups. During that year, a transformation took place unlike any I have ever seen. My patients' health improved, but something far more amazing happened. They were less depressed, happier in their relationships, and their goals shifted from not being sick to being optimally healthy. They approached their entire lives differently.

That was my initiation into the world of integrative medicine, and I have never looked back. I realized then how limited the conventional medicine I had been practicing really was. I had been treating and managing disease rather than preventing it. My medical school training prepared me to be reactive rather proactive. While this is completely appropriate in an emergency situation, it does little to help chronic conditions such as diabetes, high blood pressure and depression.

Through my experience with the Ornish study, I saw how much more there was to wellness then stents and medications. I saw how identifying and treating the underlying causes of disease such as diet, stress and lifestyle were the keys to healing not just the body, but the mind and the spirit as well. I am not saying conventional medicine is bad. I won't hesitate to prescribe a medication or a procedure when I feel it is necessary. But conventional medicine alone is not enough to achieve healing.

Holistic integrative medicine, as the name implies, integrates various therapies from many parts of the globe to achieve the most effective treatment. These may include acupuncture, diet, herbs, meditation and yes, medication. During her journey from *Heart Rending to Heart Mending* Marylou Kelly Streznewski experienced the gamut of treatments from surgery and statins to chiropractic and mantras. Her story illustrates the power of integrative medicine to not just cure, but to heal.

True health is more than the absence of disease—it is wellness of body, mind, emotions and spirit. It begins with understanding and treating the individual. Only then can we begin to heal.

Mimi Guarneri, M.D, FACC, ABIHM
Pacific Pearl, Guarneri Integrative Health Institute
La Jolla, CA
March, 2015

INTRODUCTION

WHY AM I ENTITLED TO WRITE THIS BOOK?

Think of me as a traveler returned from a long journey into far-off and exotic lands. I have a tale to tell; one which may be of help if you or a loved one should have to make this same journey, and wish for a safe return.

I will tell you what my body felt like as I experienced the difficulties of the journey. The strength of my mind and spirit was crucial in accomplishing my safe return. As on all far travels, I ingested substances which had some strange effects on me. Some of them aided, some of them threatened my return.

Did I stagger back to the everyday world to complete acceptance of my altered state? Sadly, no. Some told me, "Forget about it and go on with your life." Others claimed that certain pills could fix any problem that remained. Those who love me had to work hard to understand what had happened to me. However, I have concluded that only those who have traveled to that same strange land are able to really share and understand. For all the others, I offer my story.

How long was the journey back? Like the explorers of old, it took me over five years to find my way home. Also like those explorers, I still carry much of it with me, although I manage it better now that I have learned to understand the true nature of the journey.

I will tell my tale in prose, poems, stories and letters. There were unhappy times, even with those whose purpose was truly to help me find my way; and I will tell the truth about them. There will be at the end of my tale the stout recognition that the journey is mine—take from it what you will.

PART I

HEART RENDING

1

IF THERE WAS A KILLER STALKING...

If there was a killer stalking the women of America, murdering them at the rate of over a thousand a day, can you imagine the outcry? Well there is a killer on the loose. Its name is heart disease, and it actually does take over one thousand of our sisters, mothers, daughters, co-workers, friends and neighbors every day. I had an encounter with this killer, and survived, barely. But in the last year for which we have statistics, 400,000 women died from some form of heart disease. A woman dies somewhere in the USA every minute and a half. Every hour. Every day.

Like any other human ailment, medical science cannot save them all; but here is the most frightening statistic of all: in 64% of the cases, a woman's first encounter with heart disease is sudden death. That's right, only 36% of us even get the chance to survive. Heart disease kills six times as many women as all the cancers. Indeed, according to the author of *Dr. Suzanne Steinbaum's Heart Book*, "More women die from heart disease than all forms of cancer, chronic respiratory disease, Alzheimer's disease and accidents *combined*." [1]

Ask the average woman what is the greatest danger to her health and, according to the latest surveys, more than half of them will say breast cancer. Horrible as this disease is, and brave as its survivors obviously are, your chances of dying from it are one in thirty—for heart disease it is one in three.

Some women die of heart attacks because they don't even know they are having one. They mistake it for indigestion, take an antacid and go to bed, hoping to feel better when they wake up. They never do. They think they are developing the flu; the doctor agrees, and they go home and drop dead on the kitchen floor. Pain in the upper back and vomiting does not seem to be a heart problem; the doctor agrees, and they collapse at home and are dead before the ambulance gets there. Deep and mysterious fatigue is chalked up to the party she gave yesterday, but she dies before her husband can get her to the doctor.

She even shows up at the doctor's office with classic chest pain, which he diagnoses as an anxiety attack. Doesn't he know that an anxiety attack can be an indication of a severely leaky mitral valve?[2] He sends her home to drop dead in the shower. That's right, the doctors did not respond properly to a woman's different symptoms.

By her own admission, she can be in denial, and be lucky enough to live to tell about it. "I told myself it was indigestion, medicated myself with antacids, but I knew something was really wrong." She made it to the hospital in time.

Ask any group of mature women and you will find similar stories; these are just the ones known personally to me. Yet, there does not seem to be the same urgency surrounding the annual Red Dress campaigns that marks the wide distribution of pink ribbons and races for the cure. Can it be because only a little more than a third of us survive to tell the tale? Do we die in such large numbers because our doctors don't take our symptoms seriously, or don't recognize them as heart disease until it is too late? Is it because we don't have enough knowledge to save ourselves? How many women are told they are just getting older, working too hard, or are just too stressed?

Every medical authority, including Dr. Oz, has a checklist for prevention, most of which women know. Yes, she will agree, I should lose some weight, stop smoking, check my blood pressure and cholesterol, eat a diet full of fish and vegetables, and combat stress. But ask her to recite the special symptoms a woman may have if she is having a heart attack, and most women will draw a blank.

Lead researcher in a two-year study of these issues, Dr. Roxanna Mehran of Mount Sinai Medical Center in New York City concluded, "Women take care of their breasts and get mammograms and take care of their bones by getting bone density tests, but they often neglect their hearts." Presenting results at the American College of Cardiology in 2012, she found that the rate of heart-related death in women ages 35 to 44 is continuing to rise at the rate of 1% a year. (Reuters, March 28, 2012 *"Gynecologists urged to screen for heart disease"*)

Why is this so? According to Renee Sangrigoli, MD, a vibrant young cardiologist at the Heart Institute of Doylestown Hospital in Doylestown, Pennsylvania, and advocate for women's health, "Women may present differently than men with cardiovascular disease; making the diagnosis for the doctor can be challenging and frustrating. At times, the symptoms can be so non-specific that they are overlooked even by the patient. Women who develop heart problems are usually older than men. Since they are older, they usually have other medical problems (diabetes, high blood pressure) making them more ill on presentation."

Is this why the breast cancer campaigns have been able to reach so many women so successfully? Only a third of patients with severe heart problems survive, and most of us are in no shape to race for a cure. And even if you are fortunate, as I was, to have a brilliant surgical team save your life, what then? How do you manage recovery from the massive assault upon your body/mind/spirit in the months and years ahead?

As the survivor of eighteen months of misdiagnosis, massive heart failure and seven hours of open heart surgery; as the possessor of a replaced mitral valve, a repaired tricuspid valve, and a triple bypass; I have a very personal interest in the answers to these questions and the urge to share with others what I have learned in the years of my recovery.

In the time I spent putting my life back together I was haunted by the thought that if I had known what my own symptoms meant, I could have insisted that someone send me for heart testing. I was in and out of the offices of six different MD's in five different specialties. All of them are excellent in their fields; all of them were sympathetic; each of them had an idea about what might be wrong with me.

Nobody spotted heart disease in a 72-year old woman with high blood pressure and high cholesterol who presented the following symptoms which came and went in mysterious fashion:

Persistent unexplained severe fatigue

Anxiety, also unexplained

Heart palpitations, sleeplessness, throat pain

I noted these symptoms for the first time in March 2005, in a medical

3

notebook I started to keep. My cardiac train wreck took place December 8, 2006. Three months later, reading a newsletter published by the Friends of the Heart Center at the Doylestown Hospital where my surgery was performed, in an article written by Dr. Sangrigoli, I found the following:

Typical symptoms of heart disease include chest pain, shortness of breath and irregular heartbeats (palpitations).Women's symptoms may include:

Shortness of breath and dizziness

Flu-like symptoms

Nausea, vomiting and sweats

Unusual fatigue

Pain in upper back, jaw, neck, throat

Feelings of anxiety and malaise

I almost dropped the paper on the floor! If I had known what my own symptoms meant, I could have reminded all those doctors what they obviously knew, but were forgetting that they knew.

Nurse-researcher Dr. Jean McSweeney of the University of Arkansas Medical Services interviewed hundreds of heart attack survivors and found that 95% of them suspected something was wrong months before the actual attack. She separates the symptoms as early warnings and impending heart attack. In the first instance, get to your doctor; in the second, call 911 and get to the nearest Emergency Room.

Early-Get to Your Doctor	***Impending—Call 911***
Unusual fatigue	*Overwhelming exhaustion*
Getting winded	*Real shortness of breath*
Mood change or mild anxiety	*Sense of impending doom*
Frequent indigestion	*Terrible heartburn, nausea, vomiting*
General weakness	*No strength–like having the flu*
Chest pain, similar to a pulled muscle	*Crushing chest pain, also down right or left arm*
Headaches and periods of blurry vision	*Pain in neck, upper back, throat, jaw, both arms*
Aching in arms and hands	*Cold clammy sweat and pale skin*
Throat pain	

According to the experts, you may have any combination of these symptoms. My neighbor died because she didn't know that back pain and vomiting could be heart attack symptoms.

Dr. McSweeney found that the most frequent symptoms during a heart attack in the women she surveyed were shortness of breath, weakness and fatigue. Acute chest pain was absent in 43% of these women during their heart attack. (_http://myheartsisters.org/2012/08/27/prodromal-symptoms-pre-heart-attack_)

IF THE ABOVE LIST SOUNDS LIKE YOU, GET TO THE NEAREST HOSPITAL EMERGENCY ROOM FOR AN EVALUATION.

Over and over, on the internet, in books, news releases, e-mails and conversations the stories are the same as mine—symptoms ignored or not taken seriously, or busy women allowed to shrug off symptoms until a life-threatening crisis develops. And that is just from us survivors. How many stories from the 64% who can no longer speak? This book is dedicated to their memory.

In _A Woman's Heart, An Owner's Manual_, Drs. Eleferiades and Coulin-Glaser state, "In recent years study after study has shown that heart disease eludes detection in women, even in the hands of otherwise superbly trained and widely experienced physicians." [3]

Dr. Suzanne Steinbaum states, "Only 40-50% of primary care doctors are even aware of the cardiovascular disease prevention guidelines formulated just for women, which weren't even established until 2002." [4]

In _the Cleveland Clinic Guide to Heart Attacks_, Curtis M. Rimmerman agrees. "Incredibly, heart disease kills more women than breast cancer, yet not enough physicians have educated themselves about heart disease in women." [5]. He goes on to state, "Clinicians also fail to recognize (women's odd symptoms) as possible signs of disease." [6]

He concludes, "Women must become proactive about educating themselves and their doctors." [7]

Well intentioned campaigns focus on diet and exercise, which are extremely important. But if doctors are still having a problem connecting the dots, we women have to save ourselves by educating each other. What can you do, starting with yourself?

Dr. Sangrigoli advises, "You can't change your age, your sex or your family inheritance. (I obviously inherited the heart of my father, who died of a coronary at 54). You can quit smoking, and take the necessary steps to control your weight, blood pressure, cholesterol and diabetes."

In his *Heart Disease: An Essential Guide for the Newly Diagnosed,* Lawrence Chilnick states, "More women (38%) than men (25%) will die from heart disease in a single year…Coronary heart disease is the number-one killer of women over 25…Despite the grim well-documented stats, the threat of heart disease in women is still not universally understood…Some studies have shown that even today, less than 20% of physicians in general recognize that more women than men die of heart disease. One reason is that until recently, only 25% of the participants in all heart disease related research have been women."[8]

Clinical trials including women are slowly increasing; but so are fatalities for women in their forties. In the best of all possible worlds, every doctor, regardless of specialty, would have a poster on the wall of each examining room reminding both patient and doctor to check for heart disease. If we could make stress tests and electrocardiograms as important as mammograms, we might be able to rein in this killer.

In 2004, the American Heart Association and grass roots groups joined to create the **Go Red For Women** campaigns to educate women of all ages about the risks they face and the preventive measures they can take, if only they know about them. Too frequently women don't have the information they need before a heart attack strikes, and, as we have seen, kills them. February each year is Heart Month but once again it does not get nearly the exposure that breast cancer campaigns receive.

Both the American Heart Association and **Go Red For Women** have enormous websites filled with authentic medical information, sources for further learning, stories from survivors, recipes for a heart-healthy diet, advice for lifestyle changes, and even a powerful video called "Just a Little Heart Attack".

WomenHeart, The National Coalition for Women with Heart Disease takes a more personal approach. Facilitators, all heart attack survivors, and all trained at the Mayo Clinic, serve as volunteers who organize and host support groups for women all over the country. They also have a website filled with information and support. If you would like to see a support group in your area, contact them at http://www.womenheart.org.

You do not have to be a heart surgeon to save lives. You just have to be willing to learn about the reality of heart disease in our society and be willing to speak out about what you know. As one survivor advises, "Be a true friend and share this information with everyone you care about. You cannot do a kindness too soon, for you never know when it will be too late." This book is an effort to advance that sharing.

2

THE WORLD OF OPEN HEART SURGERY

I will take you into the world of open heart surgery from the point of view of both the surgeon and the patient. What I remember, what exactly was done to save my collapsing heart will be recounted in the appropriate forms–the surgeon's notes and the patient's poems. The surgeon's notes do not make easy reading. Indeed his secretary said, "It scared me to type them." Some of the technical medical terminology may be difficult, but where it counts, there is no mistaking the meaning.

Skilled and caring men and women had to do amazing and terrible things to my body in order to save my life. They cut me open, separated my breastbone with a bone saw; propped my chest open with clamps; hooked me up to a bypass machine to substitute for my heart and lungs. They reached into my chest cavity and laid hands on my heart and opened it up; took out the mitral valve and stitched in a new one, and repaired the tricuspid valve.

Following that, they cut open four holes in my left thigh and "harvested" the veins to use for the triple bypass. Then they undid the heart-lung machine and hoped that the repair job worked, and the tiny electrical charge which sparks our lives would catch. It didn't. Only on the third try did some part of me decide to live.

Then, of course, they had to wire my breastbone back together; sew my chest closed; put drains in my chest; IV connections for various drugs, a catheter, and unknown to me at the time, a three-day pace maker installation. Then, if I didn't succumb to infection, shock, pneumonia, or

8

various chemical imbalances, I could think about being alive again. I can write all this in prose, several years later. I could never have done it in those first months. Only poetry, or drama, can tell that story.

My experience as the patient was bizarre, psychedelic even, as it was heavily colored by various drugs. To friends and family who said, "You will have so much to write about," I replied in those early post-surgical months, that I had no desire to write about it. Indeed I did not put pen to paper at all for almost six months. We tend not to think of life-saving surgery as having bad effects. I now know that I was so "wounded" by what was done to me, that no words would come.

Current research by Bessel van der Kolk of the Boston University Medical School and the Trauma Center of Boston, has shown that severe trauma of any kind–and massive invasive surgery is severe trauma–affects the language areas of the brain. Thus when a person says they don't want to talk about what has happened, it is often that the words will not come. The value of "talk therapy" for disaster victims has come into question as we learn more about post-traumatic stress.

What finally set me back on the path was an account by another writer of her battle back from a botched double mastectomy. I went out onto my patio in the April sunshine and wrote six single-spaced pages about how I was feeling about my altered life. Only after that did the poetry begin to appear.

But that was later. Let us begin with December 7, 2006, at around...

MIDNIGHT

You are barefoot on the soft
blue of the bathroom rug when
you realize you can't breathe.
Lungs reach down, down into
space where the air should be.
It isn't.

You walk across the bedroom.
Discover you can sip the air.
Make a feeble call for husband.
No answer. Bang the wall.

He comes–plaid shirt, khakis, fear
in brown eyes below gray hair.
I think we need to go to the hospital"
Say it calmly, just as useful now
as when four babies pushed for life.

Place Medicare cards, small tan book
with children's phones, gently, in his shirt pocket.
Leave your wedding ring on the bureau.
Pull on a sweatshirt, easy to remove.

Try not to remember your father's headline:
Man Dies of Heart Attack in Doctor's Car
on Way to St. Francis Hospital.
Go carefully, carefully, down the stairs,
sipping, sipping.
Get in the car.

Marylou Streznewski is a 72 year-old white female who was admitted to Doylestown Hospital last night complaining of shortness of breath and worsening chest pain.

CHUCKLES THE CLOWN AND
AFTERNOON TEE

Trans Esophageal Echocardiogram
looks at the back of the heart

Dawn. Oxygen up my nose.
My husband sleeps on a cot.
Private room. People come and go;
ask me questions, tell me not to drink.
My husband wakes, kisses me goodbye,
says he will see me later, goes home.
The morning drags on. Test will come later.

Clack clack.
This hospital has a gentle visiting clown.
Fright wig, red bulb nose, polka dot suit, whiteface,
he says his name is Chuckles, presents me with
a small brown bear, clacks away
on his huge white shoes.
The bear regards me with stitched brown eyes.

Somehow I know. *I will call you Live-y* I tell him,
You will help me to live. The TEE cart arrives. *A bit
early for afternoon tea, I joke. Can we take the
bear?*
Of course we can't, and I climb aboard the gurney
by myself, where I will be this day, and night—by
myself.

My fashion plate cardiologist arrives, tailored suit,
frilly blouse today, assures me, *This is easy.*
You won't feel a thing. The IV goes in. I go out.
I come back to that calm voice they all use when
things are bad. I t*hink we have to do surgery.*

Then let's get it over with. I want to be home
for Christmas. The gurney rolls. I sleep.

TEE performed revealed severe mitral valve regurgitation
with a flail anterior mitral valve leaflet and prolapse of
the posterior leaflet. The patient's blood pressure
plummeted into hypotensive range. She became unstable
and was taken emergently to the cardiac catheterization
lab.

DR. B, THE CATH LAB AND ME

I awake on a cold hard surface–am I naked?
Someone is sanding my left groin; a gentle voice
is asking, *Can you feel something
in your left chest?* I can. It itch/tickles.
A balloon to go with the clown.

A large round thing descends. I see Dr. B.
The round thing goes away.

Dr. David B. performed a right and left heart
catheterization. This revealed severe multi-vessel
coronary artery disease, with severe mitral valve
regurgitation. The patient was found to have severe triple
vessel disease, and severe tricuspid valve regurgitation.
Due to cardiogenic shock, an intraaortic balloon pump
was inserted.

More voices. One says,
I'll go talk to her husband. As they slide me
onto the gurney, I call to the scrubs-clad figure
disappearing through a frosted door. *Tell him
to call the kids.*

Extensive deliberation with the patient's cardiology team
yielded a consensus to offer the patient high risk salvage
surgery. The patient had been heavily sedated for the TEE
and cath, and extensive consultation with the patient's
husband about the risks and benefits of attempting
salvage surgery occurred. The patient's husband wished
to proceed with the surgery. She was taken immediately
to the operating room.

If the Grim Reaper was skateboarding
down all those corridorsbehind us,
I didn't know it, but my gurney driver did,
because we rolled like NASCAR,

ceiling tiles, lights flying by overhead,
tall wooden doors slapping open like
the parting of the Red Sea,
under brown capital letters:
SURGICAL SUITE CARDIOLOGY.
It begins, or ends here.

"This operation has a 60-70% survival rate"

What they told the husband

In the cold watery light,
through the drug-induced stupor,
while the kindly green-robed aliens
arranged my arms in cruciform,
agreed among themselves,
You can't have too many ports,
someone made another hole in my neck.
I warned them to be careful
inserting the airway,
I don't want to come out of this in spasm.

They were probably thinking,
Lady, with what we are going to do to you,
you'll be lucky to come out of this at all.

Riding sedation into the dark,
I was completely unaware
that my brief lecture
on the proper placement of airways
might be the last words
I would ever speak.

With the patient in supine position under adequate sedation by anesthesia, adequate venous and arterial access was gained. The patient's blood pressure was low. A balloon pump was continued at 1:1, which had been placed in the cath lab. The patient was prepped and draped in routine sterile fashion from chin to toes.

THE SOUND OF KNIVES

Surgical synesthesia

Such an interesting word, K N I VE S.
The "KN" sound at the start? That is the NO!
you are too numbed to say
when they come in green robes
to open you and lay hands on your heart.

What a nice long slide the "I" makes,
as easy as the slippery path
of a scalpel down between breasts.

A small buzz for the "V" sound;
quieter no doubt than the bone saw,
which the surgeon describes
with a vertical sweep of his hand.

The Aztec priests, historians tell us,
had to be drugged to do what they did;
slicing open enemies with obsidian blades
amid the smoke of sacrifices, the screams.
Chac-Mool required all those hearts,
still beating, or he would not send the rain.
Corn would not grow. Their people would die.

The air here is clear, the bright blades
glint in the clean light.
No vicious rain-god requires this hiss,
the "S" of the plural ending, tubes
pumping blood into veins, though
some probably does splatter on the table,
the altar of this priest of life.

Opening of the sternum was performed. Simultaneously, the vein was harvested from the left leg with a mini incision approach. The left mammary artery was harvested. The left pleura was entered.

The pericardium was opened and suspended. The right heart was massively distended.

The patient was placed on cardiopulmonary bypass and cooled to 31 degrees Centigrade (87.8 Fahrenheit)

Three veins were opened. Grafts included the left internal mammary artery to a left anterior descending artery; saphenous vein graft to obtuse marginal artery; and saphenous vein graft to the right coronary artery. Good flow was noted with no leakage.

The anterior atrial groove was opened. The valve was heavily diseased with extensive myxomatous Barlow type deformity with the entire anterior leaflet prolapsing. It appeared prudent to resect this valve. The valve was resected with preservation of the posterior support structures.

There was similar pathology in the tricuspid leaflet, but with preservation of the chordal structures. Horizontal mattress sutures were placed in standard locations.

The patient was placed in deep Trendelenburg position and in temporary low flow state, and the aortic cross-clamp was released.

THE DECIDER

The lowest third of our brains,
we have in common with,
among other beings–snakes.

The prefrontal cortex makes decisions,
but it lay in anesthesia's sleep.
The limbic system manages fears and joys.
It was numb, all the gates closed.
A bypass machine ran my life.

When they cut me loose
from the surgeon's magic pump
my heart refused to start.

The patient was separated from the bypass with some
difficulty. The patient was placed back on the pump.

Once, twice, they tried, the surgeons,
they admitted later, cheering
C'mon girl, you can do it!
Third try–it caught. Some say
no anesthetic can make you deaf.
Did I hear them call me back?

After additional rest time on the pump, the patient was
then separated from the bypass with an ejection fraction
of 35-40 at least.

In that space, who decided
I would live?
Six months the question sang,
waking, dreaming; then I understood.

The ancient reptile that lives
in the bottom of the skull
did not sleep.

Eyeless, it observed.
Earless, it listened.
Voiceless, it whispered
Survive.
Survive.
Survive.

Seven #6 stainless steel wires were used to re-construct the sternum. The skin wounds were closed. Sterile dressings were applied.
Total bypass time was 5 hours; cross-clamp time was 2.8 hours. Patient was given 4 units of packed red blood cells, 15 units of platelets. The patient was transferred to the surgical intensive care unit.

THE GOSPEL ACCORDING TO
INTENSIVE CARE

On the First Day we were in Canada
for the removal of that pesky airway.
This will be fun, I said, even though
I couldn't talk. Out it slid, warm vomit
flowing down the left side of my face.

On the Second Day we were in Princeton.
A disembodied head, I watched
three cheerful nurses scrubbing
incisions I couldn't feel; teasing
the young one on my right
whose skill belied her age, they said.
They didn't know I was there.

On the Third Day I rose to consciousness–
semis whining out on the 611 Bypass,
a gray square of sky in the square window
across a large room. *"OH,* I said to no one,
This must be Doylestown. It must be dawn.

My "Lone Wild Bird" was with me all along,
words, melody floating in my head.
"Great Spirit come and rest in me," it sang,
keeping time with a wall of hissing and beeping;
a California freeway of clicking tubes
intersecting inches from my swollen right arm.

Enough electronics for a space launch,
according to my watchful son, who sat
facing them, faking confident smile,
willing the lines to stay stable, stay stable.
Don't let her die.
I slept.

And woke to white-coated voices
among the machines, debating
while I eavesdropped: *OK,
she doesn't need a pacemaker.*
Hooray! I thought. *Coumadin?*
Nobody asked me. *Coumadin? I like it,
but her cardiologist likes Plavix and aspirin.
OK, Let's keep the cardiologist happy.*

I dozed in silent agreement, until there appeared
a slender column of a man: charcoal suit,
owly glasses, center-parted brown hair,
a sweet smile, who said he was my surgeon,
apologized we hadn't met before.
I hefted a fluid-filled index finger, pointed,
slurred at him in my best drug-dopey voice,
So. You're the one who did it.

No, he corrected gently, *You did it.*
Nah, my drunk insisted, *You did it.*
Let's compromise, he smiled, *We both did it.*

The pact we made that day still holds.
We did the deed together.
Both of us are guilty
of defying the Gods.

Her 8-day postoperative course was complicated. The intraaortic balloon pump was removed on postoperative day 2. Several days of junctional rhythm required epicardial pacing. A brief episode of atrial fibrillation occurred for the first few days. Coumadin was started and then stopped.

ODE TO PERCOCET

Oh powerful painkiller, giver of vast relief
to suffering humans, I will never
forget my night with you, but
we cannot meet again–ever.

Every hour through that night I woke,
clung to my sleepless husband's hand
even while you embraced me, and begged,
Don't let them play any Beatles records!
It will screw up my machines and kill me!
Promise! and solemnly, he did.
Every hour. All night.

It was almost Christmas, so your gifts:
Holly Hobby children in red
line drawings sledding and skating
up and down the walls of my room
were fun, even with my eyes closed.

Ditto the Victoria's Secret bras and bikinis
in shades of ruby, emerald, garnet, floating,
slowly circling at the foot of my bed.

You did relieve the pain, oh Great One,
but I can't handle these one-night stands.
Darvocet must be my new romance.

The patient was placed on a fluid restriction diet and given strict sternal precautions.

THE LESSONS

On my newly conscious fourth day,
a beautiful dark-haired young
therapist smiles into my eyes.

HOW TO SIT UP
First, turn gently on your right side.
Allow the rising bed to sit you up.
Do not attempt to use the muscles
in your chest.

HOW TO STAND UP
Put legs over the side without using
your abs. She helps, this time.
Lowers bed to the floor. *Stand up*
using only your legs. Very tricky. She
holds your hands. *Now, bend your knees*
only a little, three times, and you can go
back to bed. Reversing of course,
lessons one and two.

MANAGING FOOD
Now, you must sit in a chair for meals.
Knee-bending is into a chair, legs only;
beware the catheter. You are weak.
The nurse is kind when she says,
If you want the milk, you must
open the carton yourself. I get it.
They want me stronger every day.

REMOVING CHEST DRAINS
For this, we must rehearse. Then for each,
counting, breath-holding, nurse pulls one,
then two, then three. Lying flat for twenty
minutes–*No moving at all.*

TAKING A SHOWER
They know on day six that I can.
I'm not so sure. We walk to the
sit-down shower, my IV and me;
I even wash my hair.

TAKING A WALK
*The required course is twice
around the Cardiac Section.*
My favorite evening nurse
bribes me with a cup of tea,
my IV and me.

CLIMBING STAIRS
Would you like to go home on Saturday?
Not before you climb the stairs.
So out to the fire stairs we go, leaving
IV behind. Daughter on one side,
nurse on the other, we learn a clever little
*Flex-your–foot-and-ankle-do-not-use-your
abs-or-chest* routine–it works. Lessons
complete, I graduate to home!

The patient is discharged with pleural fluid in her left chest. All things considered, Mrs. Streznewski did remarkably well.

3

COMING HOME–
CLEAN AND HELPLESS, WEAK AND WEEPY

On December 18, after 8 days of treatment, they wheeled me down to the hospital entrance on a cold sunny Saturday morning and began the process of packing me into the back seat of our SUV. Yes, the back seat, where I was required to ride until the doctors said otherwise. I was weak and shaky as they settled me in, and they packed a nice fluffy bed pillow between me and the seat belt.

Riding home through the winding streets of our suburban neighborhood, it all felt strange, as if I had been away for a very long time. At the same time it all looked unchanged. I guess I expected, given the drama I had experienced, it would somehow all be different. The sight of home was most welcome.

I had planned exactly where I would stay, in a recliner which I had asked to be moved from the living room to my husband's study, so I would not be isolated. Like the best-laid plans of you-know-who, it proved too uncomfortable at first, and I wound up monopolizing his soft leather sofa instead, propped on pillows and wrapped in an afghan.

Norman Cousins, who should know, says in *The Healing Heart: Antidotes to Panic and Helplessness*, that, "Continuing progress toward recovery requires: emotional and psychological factors, family support, proper nutrition, proportionate exercise, and a way of life that looks forward to each day." [9]

"The bathroom must be scrubbed from top to bottom every day to avoid the slightest chance of Mom getting an infection."

Thus read just one of the directives to her three siblings which my eldest daughter Marina composed and gathered into a large three-ring notebook. Having worked as an EMT in Washington, DC, she was well-qualified to supervise the first days of my at-home care, as the family prepared for Christmas. And given that I still had unhealed incisions in chest and legs, as well as three seeping chest drains, cleanliness precautions were quite sensible.

That great blue notebook became the Bible for my care. There were med schedules, fluid limit charts, and a large amount of material from the hospital. There were directions for putting on clothes without raising my arms (a no-no with a re-wired breast bone), foods to eat and avoid, diet, wound care, when to call the doctor, and a week-by-week chart of when I could expect to resume normal activities.

Given my helpless state, the use of the antiseptic bathroom to bathe me was a humbling and loving experience. The room was warmed to steam-bath status; my daughter stripped to her underwear, and helped me, entirely naked, into a sliding shower chair and washed oh so gently. In those moments of intimacy and very special caring, I thought of harems where women cared for each other, and remembered that this was the same room where I washed these same children.

I was helpless in many other ways. Because of the chest drains and my wired-together sternum, getting in and out of bed was a production, not to be attempted alone. Bathroom need at 3:00.a.m.? Wake up husband. Roll carefully onto right side. Husband helps to lift me to vertical; legs come over the edge of the bed. Stand up, using only legs—I learned it in the hospital. Escort to bathroom and special raised john seat—be lowered into place. Return trip. The hardest part, lowering me down into bed again. Husband permanently injured tendons as a result.

Dressing a helpless adult is nothing like Mommy dressing a child. I wore tops that could button and pants that could be donned sitting down. The most fun was the socks. Raising four kids, I put socks on thousands of resistant little feet, but Husband lacked my extensive experience. It was for him a lengthy task; for me frustration

In spite of the fluid restrictions, eating was fun. Knowing that a more limited cardiac diet was in my future, I appreciated my surgeon's partner, a sensible European gentleman, giving me the following permission: "You have had a tremendous shock to your system, and you need to be nourished to get well. For the next six weeks you should eat anything you like." And I did.

Only much later would I fully realize how being completely taken care of helped me through those difficult first weeks. Each of my four offspring, two boys and two girls, took a week out of their busy lives to take care of me and their still-in-shock father.

Next in line after Marina was our West Point graduate son, Andrew. Handy at anything needing repair, he also did military-standard housekeeping, prompting me to exclaim, "I want to keep you here; you would be the perfect butler!" Another of his useful people skills was helping to smooth things over when his parents' frayed emotions and nerves resulted in angry words.

Tom Junior is a modern dad of two boys. He came down from Maine to continue the stream of excellent housekeeping, help with cooking and overall support. By now the "bathing assistance" chores had been taken over by my husband, much to the relief of the two boys.

Finally there came Alex, mother of two girls, attorney, great cook and deep believer that life should be fun. She kept up with her job via our computer, produced gourmet meals, and ferried me to my doctor's appointment, in the back seat and still packed with pillows. She replied to my question about the odd route she was taking to get home with, "'It is time you got out of the house. (It was now the end of January) So unless you kick and scream, we are going to Starbucks for your favorite chai and a pastry." And so we did.

What did my family do with this clean and helpless person as we moved on toward Christmas? There would be no tree, despite my pleas. "You are the Christmas present; it's all we need," I was told.

The presents were stacked in a pyramid in front of the living room window. I was too weak to pick up a package containing glass coasters as a gift. My children made our traditional Christmas Eve and Christmas dinners. The latter was not very merry as I burst into tears in the middle of it.

In talking with other heart event survivors (more about the necessity of doing that in a later section) I realized how much post-op pain I was spared after coming home, although my single problem with pain was quite enough.

Recall the reference to my "arms in cruciform" in the poem "**This Operation Has a 60% Survival Rate**". My previously injured right trapezius (back) muscle had a delayed reaction to being in that position for seven hours. It spasmed on Christmas night. The pain was excruciating, and it took both my husband and my physical therapist son-in-law just to get me into bed. Several days of heat and the application of electrical stimulation with a TENS device calmed things down. It is a chronic problem which I have had to learn to manage.

On December 26, my surgeon declared that there was no more fluid in my lungs and, "You look as good from the x-rays on the inside as you do on the outside." I could fire him, he told me with a smile, because his work was finished. As the days moved on there was the visiting nurse, then the physical therapist who gave me a set of gentle exercises and then said, "Get your coat, so we can go for a walk." Wrapped up like a terrorist, I walked and chatted with him in the January sun.

I was then directed to walk for 20 minutes twice a day. Since it was January, most of my walking was done in the house: all around the first floor, up the steps and all around the bedrooms and my study, listening for the oven timer to set me free. To relieve the boredom I got out my old Walkman and donned earphones. The cheerful discs I selected led to dancing, which did get a little out of hand, but I knew I was making progress.

My days were spent thus: the getting-dressed routine and then breakfast, after which I climbed into my "cocoon"—the recliner where I wrapped myself in a quilt and slept. Exercises and walking were followed by lunch and reading. My reading was carefully selected to be light and/or amusing. Those of a literary bent may appreciate that I actually read and enjoyed Proust. *Remembrance of Things Past* was so spaced-out and dreamy that it provided ideal amusement. I also had a lot of time to think about what had been placed inside my chest.

THE CALF

Mitral valve replacement 6900ptfx
Tissue source: calf

I think about him often; every day it seems.
In my fantasy world he nuzzles his mother
for milk, enjoys a few sky-blue days of animal joy
kicking up his tiny hooves in a grassy field,
before the Two-Leggeds come and lead him
into a strange barn that moves away,
away out of his dumb mother's sight,
to the ritual slaughter that harvests
his heart to rescue mine.

It only starts with a calf, my surgeon tells me.
It's processed in a lab, reminding me once again
that the cold precision only science knows
gave me this mitral valve, saved my life.

But I need to go on believing
that inside these ticking alien
cells keeping me alive
there is a mother's warmth,
sunlight in a sapphire sky,
and delicious grass.

Each day in the later afternoon, I began a routine which I follow sometimes even now. Using a collection of relaxation tapes, notably one called "Tibetan Meditation Music" I combined sound therapy with imaging for a session of serious relaxation.

A NOTE: As I tell my story in prose and poems, I will mention the healing modalities which helped me, but a detailed discussion of the value of each will come later, in **Heart Mending**.

Dinner was followed by being required to laugh. My Christmas present from my husband was the entire collection of the British sit-com "Are You Being Served?" It lasted for many healing evenings. Almost every source I consulted advocated the value of laughter in the healing process.

My favorite appears in Norman Cousins' book, *The Healing Heart Antidotes to Panic and Helplessness*. He quotes a 17th century physician, Thomas Sydenham, who said, "The arrival of a good clown exercises more beneficial influence upon the health of a town than twenty asses laden with drugs." Big Pharma take note.

Each evening of the early weeks featured more indoor walking, and was followed by the bath production, then the getting into bed production and sleep. Each night I inched a wee bit over to ease my insatiable desire to lie on my left side, hesitant to use my wounded body the way I used to. Finally getting there was a triumph.

Then of course there came the firsts: bathing and dressing alone (even socks!), riding in the front seat of the car without the pillows; actually driving; beginning to help with the cooking.

When You First Come Home

So, Dear Fellow Surgery Survivor (and family), what should you do in the early weeks, as your bones and tissues begin to knit themselves back together, to begin the healing of mind, body and spirit as one?

Studies have shown that training both patient and family to follow a careful regimen of care in the early weeks can greatly reduce complications and readmissions, as well as speed recovery. An NBC News report (9/2/1013) states that a study shows that hospital-to-home focus may reduce readmissions.

Based on my own experience, I am going to presume to give you some reminders and some advice:

1. Listen to your doctor's instructions and follow the self-care provisions exactly, especially those concerning your wired-together breastbone.

2. Take the medicines prescribed and keep in close touch with your doctor as to how they are working out. It is more likely than not that they will have to be adjusted several times over the coming weeks.

3. Do whatever exercises you are directed to do by physical therapists or visiting nurses *no matter how boring they are*. I was required to walk for 20 minutes twice a day. It was January so I walked in the house–talk about boring!

4. *Laugh* every day. Every evening my family sat me down to watch "Are You Being Served?" and have my dose of laughing for the day; use whatever makes you laugh.

5. Be patient with being somewhat helpless. I needed help in bathing, getting dressed, getting in and out of bed, waking my husband when I had to use the bathroom during the night. Having someone else put on my socks was an adventure. Being bathed by my two daughters recalled the times spent in the same bathroom as I bathed them as children.

6. To the degree that you can, avoid upsetting TV shows, magazine articles, novels, and stay off the social media for a while.

In the weeks when I did little more than eat, sleep, read, take naps and visit my cardiologist (an adventure with pillows to cushion the seat belt over my chest) I read old potboilers from high school.

More Independence

As time goes on, you can dress yourself and shower alone, although the first time performing the latter I was a bit nervous and needed someone nearby. You can turn over in bed and relax a bit more for better sleep. My sensible doctor allowed only a night or two of sleeping pills when I came home, although I had plenty of pain meds.

If you are fortunate enough to have a hospital with a good cardiac rehab program, *do not fail to attend on a regular basis*. Study after study has confirmed that those who follow a cardiac rehab exercise program of whatever kind, have a much better survival rate. And you haven't come through all this to quit now, have you?

Speaking Of Survival

I recall hearing Dr. Andrew Weil on a radio program where the interviewer challenged him to explain why, in a book called *Healthy Aging*, the whole first chapter is devoted to the fact that we are all going to die. Reminding myself of how Dr. Weil answered that challenge is one of the things that gets my lazy body off to the gym, or out into the garden, or even a short walk after dinner.

He explained that first, we are all going to die, and that must be accepted. Barring unexpected disasters, we can choose to live an active, healthy-as-we-can life right up until our body gives out. Or we can be inactive and unhealthy and wind up wasting away for several miserable years. In his experience, Dr. Weil related, the people who make the first choice (as best they can) "live 'til they die" and their passing is usually less prolonged and less agonizing. He spends the rest of his interesting book showing the reader how to make the first choice.

You may have noticed by now that I received excellent advice and care from the hospital and my doctors, for my body—but not much was said about my mind, emotions and spirit. My physical body was healing and they were pleased. Even I did not know that I had much more work to do, and that I would have to educate myself to do it

I began 12 weeks of Cardiac Rehabilitation at the hospital's facility. Here we did stretches, exercised on stationary bikes, treadmills and elliptical trainers while wearing heart monitors to track our progress. The exercises were mostly boring, but the atmosphere was caring and positive. I teased the therapists that they must pump something special into the air because just walking in the door made me feel better. I would realize only later that the only thing they pumped in was their own positive energy, and it changed the way the air felt. Energy work of various kinds has helped me on my journey and will have its own section later.

Sharing The Train Wreck

As a new spring began to appear, the Newsletter of the International Women's Writing Guild arrived with a note from member Alice Orr, who had survived a botched double mastectomy and had us all fearing for her life. Her use of the train wreck image to describe her experience, the same one I was using, opened the gates to writing again, and allowed me to put down my thoughts about my altered life in a letter to her. Then I was able to begin to write the poems.

Dear Alice;

Reading your note in the IWWG Newsletter struck a familiar chord for me. Interesting how each of us used the image of a train wreck to describe illness invading our lives. In my case, the collapse of my (misdiagnosed) heart in December of 2006 is referred to as a cardiac train wreck. I still marvel at a surgeon with the nerve to replace a mitral valve, repair a tricuspid valve and do a triple bypass on a 72-year-old lady!

I write to you in great sympathy for the frustration of "cannot" when "can" has always been taken for granted—as in "I can put on my own socks and take a shower by myself." Being washed and dressed like a child for weeks after open heart surgery was so distressing. Now as I put on my tights and socks(!) for the exercises which I will do for the rest of my life, I try to remind my complaining self, "Remember when you couldn't put on your own socks?"

I try, as I'm sure you do, to be glad I'm still here. However, wandering through a supermarket filled with things I am no longer allowed to eat, I sometimes come close to tears. The person whose two favorite things are fat and salt is not a happy camper.

I worry about how long I may live. I can't get a real answer about how long replaced heart valves last. "Yours is state-of-the-art, too new, we don't know," they tell me. The worry has led to a wide variety of spiritual reading, from our own Mechi Garza, to the Dalai Lama, to the comfort of certain poets.

Though I am sure that long term, although the fear picture attached to cancer is different, it is difficult to get others to understand that it is always there. Case in point: A gentleman I know from the gym where I do cardiac rehab just revealed on Friday (when someone asked him how his summer went) that he had a large cancer removed from his cheek in August and, "My wife does not understand that this has turned my world upside down." We shared the idea of the fear that is always there, lurking beneath even the happy moments.

Another phenomenon that haunts some heart patients, including myself, is a weird inability to accept good news. The cardiologist says, "You are my champion patient!" and you still wonder...but you are so right in saying that the "cannots" are the worst part of life's derailments. One tries not to remember "before the surgery," but it comes up all the time.

The question keeps arising, "Where can I get more energy?" Ole Man Fatigue, or is it Ole Lady? ambushes me almost daily. Way-back-when, when I was juggling four kids, a big house, a full time job and graduate school, my motto was, "I'll sleep when I'm dead." I copied it from Rosalind Russell, who died very bravely of cancer. I would get by on four or five hours of sleep. Now the equipment I have to work with requires nine or ten of the precious 24 if I am to function at all.

And that is part of the way back, though I admit to resenting every step. I am allowed to do most things I love, gardening, writing and the required exercises, if I do them in small segments. Example: Twenty-five minutes of seated weed-pulling and five minutes of light raking did me in this morning, meaning a sedentary second half of the day. I am learning to plan my life around my "allowance" of energy, like a householder coping with a small budget.

I have not at all mastered the acceptance of the fact that I can no longer tackle housecleaning, furniture moving, or "Let's paint the dining room,"—not ever. If my do-it-yourself self ever finds peace, I will be one enlightened old lady!

I am planning my first adventure in going away from home all by myself. I am driving an hour and a half to the North Jersey mountains for the four-day Dodge Poetry Festival. It is held in a restored historic village and so involves lots of walking as well as sitting in workshops and panels. It is a feast I wouldn't miss, but the careful regulation of my strength is a somewhat daunting prospect. I will stay at a nearby motel, alone, but my afternoon nap will have to take place in the festival parking lot in my Blazer.

As to writing, there are several considerations. At first I was annoyed at those who said, "Oh, you have so much to write about." I have had no desire to write about what I have been living through for many months. But as a direct result of reading about your cancer battle in the IWWG Newsletter, what I am willing to say about my surgery began to pour forth, first in this letter, and then in a series of poems. The first four became six and then more as I wrote about this struggle.

Stumbling toward the light is also helped immensely by nature. The light in this late afternoon has sprinkled through the pine trees next door. Beauty is a great healer. And I am learning, after the great train wreck, to manage here along this smaller-gauge track. Maybe it's just a monorail now. I almost said, "For now." I still haven't learned—maybe I'm not supposed to.

All the best,
Marylou

4

RE-ENTERING THE WORLD

A Question Of Pills

In the several months after my surgery we were still adjusting and changing my blood pressure meds. My regular cardiologist was not available, so another member of the practice, a very competent doctor, saw me. After we had settled on the blood pressure prescription, he asked how I was doing otherwise. I mentioned that aside from what I considered minor problems with depression and anxiety, I was doing fine. He immediately became very concerned, and indicated that in the first year especially, this can be a serious concern.

He then urged me to see my primary doctor for a prescription to calm me. "You need to be on something, and he is good at this. Don't let this go." I thanked him with no intention of heeding his advice, and solving my problems with a pill bottle. Indeed, when I related this to my regular cardiologist, she agreed that I probably didn't need pills. She knew that I was doing yoga, listening to meditation tapes and recommended a walk in the Spring sunshine if I was feeling blue. "You're into all that natural stuff; you're not the pill type," she smiled.

This episode begins to illustrate some of the problems I was to encounter in my efforts to combine the best of all healing possibilities with conventional medicine. First, for all his very real caring and skill, the other doctor did not know me as well as the person who had seen me through the surgery.

Second, for all his knowledge, he could only offer me pills when, as I learned in years of searching, there are so many other ways to calm fears and soothe anxieties.

Dealing With Fear

By May I could drive across the river to have lunch with old friends. Nervous at being alone and farther from home than I had been since December, I felt really accomplished as I pulled into the restaurant parking lot. Like literally hundreds of times since then, I asked myself why I had been afraid. It would be a long time before I understood my own fear.

And an even longer time before I understood some strange symptoms. You will have noticed that I received world-class care from a host of caring people—for my body. But no one warned me about dealing with my emotions, mind, and spirit. Why, for example, would I enter the kitchen, say good morning to my husband, and burst into tears? While driving my husband to the doctor (he had injured his arm helping me in and out of bed in the early days) we were discussing an upcoming visit from our grandchildren, and all I could think of were problems that might arise. I banged the steering wheel and exclaimed, "Why must I always be so fearful and negative? Why?" And why would I awake on some mornings almost flattened with fear and nameless anxiety? Finding the answers led me to research on Post Traumatic Stress Syndrome, because, as Dr. Memet Oz has said, "We now understand that surgery is controlled trauma."

Cardiac Rehab–For Life

Also in May I graduated to Phase III of the hospital's Cardiac Rehab program at the local wellness center and gym, to a program supervised by a physical therapist. I will be there for the rest of my life. Exercise is that important. Here there were more machines, a pool, and access to other classes, especially yoga. I had never thought of myself as a gym rat, but again the staff created an air so pleasant and supportive that it helped the workouts.

I had done conventional Hatha Yoga for many years, and therapeutic yoga in the months of my misdiagnosis. Now I asked my doctors for advice about returning to it. And here again, we see the problem which exists in so many phases of modern medical care. None of my doctors, caring as they were, could advise me, because they knew nothing about yoga. Fortunately, the Wellness Center created a class specifically for Rehab patients, which offered yoga in a chair. It is a form which is increasingly popular for anyone with limitations from surgery, joint replacement or other injuries.

In addition, I was able to return to my massage therapist for regular visits; for work on the trapezius muscle which spasmed on Christmas night. I was fortunate that my knowledge of various healing modalities and their regular use was already in place in my life before my cardiac train wreck.

I had done yoga for over twenty years; massage for three or four, and acupuncture for a year or so. I had experimented with various types of meditation, relaxation, and meditation tapes as well. I had approached each one with the same skeptical question, "Does this stuff work?" and I found that the answer was "Yes."

Travel

June brought the biggest challenge so far. Could I make my annual trip to the conference of the International Women's Writing Guild at Skidmore College, a five-hour drive from my home in Pennsylvania? Previously, I had been the driver for a friend; now she arranged to transport me.

A week away from home, away from my doctors, lots of walking, taking care of myself completely? I was afraid, but determined to go. My cardiologist said, "Have fun!" If she was confident, why was I so afraid? Truth to tell, I was afraid most of the time.

To give myself confidence, I did several things which I still do each time I travel any distance outside the range of my local hospital. First, I purchased a Medi-Alert bracelet. They come in a variety of type, bracelets and lockets. Mine opens to reveal my medical info, doctor's number and allergies. At all times, I carry the cards identifying the manufacturer and type of my replaced mitral valve and repaired tricuspid valve, in my wallet right next to my Medicare card.

For longer trips like the one to the conference at Skidmore, I have assembled a summary of my multiple medical conditions and my meds, which I place in plain sight in my hotel or dorm room, and carry in my briefcase. It helps to ease the fear of being taken ill away from home.

At the Skidmore conference I received lots of healing hugs, and praise for doing so well. All the sources I consulted on mind/body medicine agreed that emotional support, including hugs, can result in lowering of blood pressure, and easing of anxiety and depression. I was also able to speak to the women about the warning signs of heart disease. When I reminded them that their chance of dying from a heart attack is one in four, there was an audible gasp from the audience of four hundred women.

There Is Always Something

After Skidmore I was sailing! A week on my own had proved that my energy limitations could be worked with. My "numbers" (cholesterol) had my cardiologist proclaiming that I was her ideal patient. My daily visits to my mother in a local nursing home were going well. Now that I could lie comfortably on my stomach, I returned to regular massage therapy. I was finishing my novel and beginning to work on the poems found in this book.

Then came a cascade of events which I prided myself on handling well. Little did I suspect what lay ahead. First came cataract surgery—two more "implants," these in my eyes. After 60 years of having close up vision, which allowed me to function most of the time without my glasses, needing glasses only for distance and things like driving, my orientation to the world was reversed. The implants gave me distance vision and took away my ability to read, to see my own body; I now wore glasses virtually all the time. I am still adjusting.

Two weeks after that, my 100-year-old mother fell and broke her hip, and with the marvels of medical science, she was able to undergo successful surgery to fix her hip. However, there followed a six-week ordeal of her mental derangement while the after-effects of the anesthetic wore off, and she refused all forms of physical therapy.

Not surprisingly, September featured my third attack of diverticulitis, an intestinal inflammation notoriously brought on by stress. With a caring and understanding surgeon, we agreed to put off a colon resection until January, so that I could have a nice Christmas, unlike the previous one. To help me manage the pain and discomfort of waiting, I turned to my Chinese acupuncturist and was able to manage until after the holidays. Here again we see another form of alternative medicine which proved extremely helpful in my healing process.

Recovery from the colon surgery (a laparoscopic procedure) was smooth and by March I was back at my regular exercise level and feeling fine. But my mother wasn't. Despite a flu shot, she contracted the flu in February, and began a long slow bedridden decline. I visited her daily at a nursing home near my house. She celebrated her 101st birthday and died in early June. Her memorial service was comforting to all of us in its informality and warmth.

Four days later I headed to Skidmore again and the comforting arms of my writing sisters. This time, walking around the campus was tiring. Ominously tiring, because in the weeks that followed, my hip and back pain worsened. I began to be unusually tired and neither massage nor acupuncture seemed to help. So after 18 months of taking statins without incident, I began what I have come to call...

5

THE BATTLE OF THE STATINS

I Am Not A Medical Authority

It went on from June 2008 to June 2009, and to tell the truth, it isn't over yet. I cannot caution the reader enough that I am not a medical authority. I can only relate what happened to me. None of what follows should be taken as advice on your own condition. Each person must consult his or her medical professional before starting or stopping any medication or treatment. You will find that his section weaves in and out between what was happening to me and what I was learning from my research—somewhat like the back-and-forth with the poems and the surgical notes.

For 18 months, I had been taking the smallest dose of Vytorin which the pharmaceutical company recommends, 20mg, with no ill effects. I didn't know then that many patients actually need only 10 mg—or even 5mg—but only a few drug companies make these small doses available. I also didn't know that around 18 months was the time that many other patients, who had been doing fine, began to see side effects.

I returned from the Skidmore conference with my knees and hips sore—ominously sore. I blamed it on too much walking and assumed I just needed some rest. After all, everything was going so well, wasn't it...? Well, there was the whole thing with these waves of anxiety that would come out of nowhere. I would sometimes wake in the morning feeling worried, but not knowing what I was worried about.

Or there were days when the world looked like a very dark place indeed, and I was terribly depressed. Then there were incidents of putting a negative, fear-based interpretation on the simplest everyday events. Getting in the car, I would picture myself in an accident. Watching my husband walk out to the mailbox, I would wonder, "What if he falls?" Riding in an elevator would prompt, "What if it gets stuck?" My eldest daughter finally lost patience and scolded, "Why must you always be so negative?" And there was the question that I now know so many others have asked lying alone in the dark, "Am I going crazy?"

On through July the joint pains persisted, and I recorded in my diary that I could not use the treadmill at cardiac rehab. I was more tired than usual, and I was having trouble focusing my eyes. I have a muscle imbalance in my right eye, aggravated by five hours on the bypass machine, and it has always been my indicator that I am getting sick.

By August I noted an episode while out shopping in our little town. Finishing up some errands, I headed across the street to the dry cleaners. Suddenly there was this funny feeling in my legs, as if the muscles have turned to mush and didn't want to work. Here is where I began to research muscles, and found that statins may affect several enzymes in muscle cells that are responsible for muscle growth. The effects of statins on these cells may be the cause of muscle aches. And unexplained weakness out of nowhere?

Pain and weakness where increasing in September, and I recalled an NPR broadcast I heard several years ago that stuck with me. Reports were coming in indicating that patients on these new statin drugs were complaining of aches and pains, even though their tests of liver function were normal. The question was raised even then, were heart patients doomed to simply live with aches and pains for the rest of their lives?

The scene: October in my ophthalmologist's waiting room. I run into a fellow poet whom I hadn't seen in a long time and we catch up on each other's lives. When I mention my battle with the statins, he says, "Oh yes, my wife is taking them and they are making her so sick. We don't know what to do; the doctor insists that she take them."

The tech calls me in. As part of the history she is taking, I must mention the problems with statins, she says, "Oh statins. My poor father has refused to continue to take them. He says he will not spend the rest of his life with these miserable aches and pains."

The doctor completes his exam and wishes me luck. I remark that I will be fine if the statins don't get me, and remind him of the MDs I have read about who want to put them in the drinking water. His voice dripping with sarcasm, he says, "Of course, we should give them to everybody. They'll make us live longer!" and grinning, he goes out the door.

Researching Statins

I was cutting my exercise sessions shorter and shorter and was still in pain. I began reading websites and getting books from the library to research statins. I found two books to be especially helpful: *What You Must Know about Statin Drugs & Their Natural Alternatives*, by Jay S. Cohen, MD, and *Reverse Heart Disease Now*, by Stephen T. Sinatra, MD and James C. Roberts, MD. A series of others are in the list at the back of the book.

To begin, both authors took great pains to acknowledge that statins help to save lives. However, they also discussed openly their findings that many patients (up to one-third in some cases) were having serious joint pain, fatigue and mental/emotional problems, including memory loss. What could be done?

Cohen emphasizes that statin dosage must be tailored to each individual patient dependent on how much reduction is needed, as well as how the patient reacts to statins. His solution is to start small. How small? Very small—5mg, in some cases. He actually gives a series of charts for the major statin brands showing how the percentage of reduction can be keyed to the size of the dose.[10] This is followed by an entire chapter of evidence-based information on the effectiveness of lower doses of statins. According to Cohen, once the desired level is achieved, anything more is an overdose—and, most importantly, the source of many undesirable side effects.

At the same time I began doing research on the Internet, sticking only to what seemed to be reliable sources like the prestigious Cleveland Clinic and the Mayo Clinic. On the Mayo Clinic website I was assured that there was no evidence that statins could affect memory. Muscle and joint pain? Cut back on your exercise. Pain management? Do not use over the counter pain relievers as they are not very effective for this kind of pain. I must also note that down the right side of this page of advice runs a rolling commercial for Lipitor. At the bottom of the page one is informed that the selling of this ad space serves to support the website.

My cardiologist suggests a switch to Crestor. I decline, having read all kinds of negative reports, and noting that it is the strongest of the statins. If the statins are causing my problems, why would I want to take more? But who am I supposed to believe?

Who Can I Trust?

By November I am too tired for aerobic exercise at all, and struggling to do my yoga class. There are pains and fears galore. How can I make a life out of this? Dr. Sangrigoli advises taking Vytorin until the end of December. This is the doctor whose quick thinking got me into the OR with a top surgeon who saved my life. How can I not trust her advice?

By now it hurts to walk up every one of the 22 steps from cardiac rehab to street level. I have pain in my wrist, hand and arm. The pains in my hips are terrible. Could this be sciatica? At the end of December, my cardiologist states emphatically that the pains are not from the statins.

A January visit to a neurologist finds no sciatica, nor any problem with discs. "Could be bursitis of the trocanter, the spot where all the muscles come together over the hip joint." He recommends massage, which I am already doing for the pain in my shoulder, and suggests I see an orthopedist for my knee. The list of doctors is getting long—it will get longer.

My lower right abdomen is sore, so it is off to the gynecologist for various tests. I have sonograms of ovaries and kidneys, a mammogram, and a dexascan which finds mild osteoporosis of the left hip and lumbar spine, but not enough to cause this kind of pain.

The orthopedist is an old friend who did MRI's of the shoulder and knee and he said, "Saw no changes from the original injuries." By this time I had given up Cardiac Rehab completely—not a good thing for a heart patient like myself. He prescribed physical therapy to try and get some muscle strength back.

Before leaving I asked my old friend, "Do you have other patients who have these mysterious pains which nobody can seem to identify, but who just all happen to be on statins?" He gave me a slow smile and a one word answer, "Lots." His advice: "The smallest dose you can possibly manage," a reflection of Dr. Cohen's advice.

Tired and depressed, but determined to learn anything I could, I attended a lecture on statins by a local cardiologist. It featured lots of graphs, and a bit of a whirl about mortality rates, what the graphs actually prove, etc. He did admit that the claims for statins should be taken with a grain of salt; that they are not for everyone; and that there have been some memory and confusion problems—which at that time Big Pharma did not admit.

Most poignant of all was the question from an elderly gentleman in the audience who asked, "Well, if they are supposed to be keeping me from another heart attack, does that mean that I have to spend the rest of my life feeling like I have the flu?" The doctor advised him to ask his cardiologist to consider a change of dose or a change in statin.

TO GAIA—THE GREAT MOTHER

When she asked,
"Child, why are you crying?"

There are tears that need to be cried, Mother,
to honor the things we grieve for.
The party's almost over and we cannot dance
the way we used to. We so loved the dancing—
moving our bodies, energized by love.

Now The Numbers tells us that to live at all,
we must take the pills, drink the potions,
live as ones who do not dance but stagger—
pain in the body, fog in the mind.
They say we do not know our place,
our house, our home, our bodies
where we have lived so long,
our cells reborn ten times or more.

The Numbers do not tell the truth.
Our mitochondria know-
the life force lives within their walls,
says "NO" to chemical invaders.
But The Numbers insist
We are large. You must obey.

Stalking through the universe, The Numbers tell us
they know what living is. Behind placebo masks,
they boast of being double-blind.
We see with eyes we own. We weep, Mother,
on the days it seems we must bow to our masters.
We do not know what else to do when they intone,
You will have another Event, guaranteed.
Even death, they claim they can measure.

February 20, 2009, was an important milestone in taking responsibility for my own care. I took my massage therapist out to lunch. Mary Ellen is legally blind. When we left the restaurant, I could not remember how to drive to her house, less than a mile away across a town I have lived in for over 40 years! Eventually, after some aimless meandering, I found my way without her knowing I had been lost. But I knew. And I had to ask myself, if I can't be trusted to find my way home, can I no longer be allowed out alone?

Both Drs. Cohen and Sinatra were openly discussing memory problems they had seen in patients on statins. According to an internet article from *Scientific American* "It's Not Dementia. It's your Heart Medication: Cholesterol Drugs and Memory," (2/10/11), hundreds of people have registered complaints with the FDA, and experts are starting to believe that a certain percentage of patients may be at risk.

The article goes on to explain the connection between cholesterol drugs and the brain. Actually one-fourth of the body's cholesterol is found in the brain, where it plays a vital role in the formation of neuronal connections, the vital links that underlie memory, cognition, quick thinking and rapid reaction times. A drug that affects such an important pathway is bound to have some adverse reactions, says Ralph Edwards, the former director of the World Health Organization's drug-monitoring center.

SWISS CHEESE

I am barreling along at the speed of thought
pausing only to construct the next idea, when
I look into the jar of Trail Mix I am opening
and find
empty
space,
a hole
inside
my head
I see
a shape:
tan
ribbed
oval.

Tiny
panic
until
I can
say:

almond
almond,
this is
an almond.

Repeat.
Almond.
For next time.

Kitchen again.
Husband across table.
I forgot to fill the...

Point.
Frown.
Struggle.

Tiny
panic
until
I can
say
ice cube trays.

Six PM on NPR.
Prairie Home Companion.
I really enjoy...

Nine twenty-five PM.
It comes.
Garrison Kiellor.

I have
holes
in my brain
like
Swiss Cheese.

While I worried about my memory, there were more tests to find the cause of my problems. They included a heart monitor for a week, a nuclear stress test which was, "As good as it was in November 2007." The gynecologist wants to check calcium levels and some other blood work. There is a problem with my parathyroid which could require surgery. I am seeing an endocrinologist and may have to see a surgeon at the University of Pennsylvania. All these doctors! We are up to nine, so far, and no answers.

I am beginning to feel like a laboratory specimen! My primary says, "Your case may pique the interest of the surgeon at Penn because it's so odd."

POO! "I do not exist to pique anybody's interest. The issue is my pain and my personhood!" a comment I kept to myself. Testing for the parathyroid condition involves two x-rays where I must lie still for 45 minutes each, and in the end there does not seem to be a problem.

Everyone continues to want to "try things," anything but blame the statins. They don't buy my memory problems, but my cardiologist agrees to 14 days off the statins and then I must take Pravachol (another brand) 20mg every other day. My diary entry notes: "The more I read, the more I understand that I have been damaged by these pills! I am not sure the doctor realizes how long I should be off them to get valid results. Three days and already I feel better!"

I tease the 14 days out to 21 days and I get back on my exercise machines, my muscles and joints are recovering in physical therapy. I need less rest, and I am very conscious of a clear mind. I have done more writing in the past 21 days than I have in months. I start Pravachol reluctantly, (I'm still trying to be a good patient and listen to the doctors) and within three days the same old stuff is back.

Taking Charge

April and May are simply a dance of phone calls between the cardiologist, and my primary, who do not agree on how to proceed. Eventually, I stop the Pravachol and decide that I am taking charge of, and responsibility for, my own fate, my own health, my own life, my own death, but the choices would be mine.

THE REVENANT

A person who returns as a spirit after death; a ghost.

I remember him dressed all in white
in the painting, a ghostly sailor
washed in the dusty antique mirror
of Andrew Wyeth's mind and vision.

I wonder about my Self.
Am I new after near death?
A ghost?
Somebody died on that table.
What white-clothed revenant
was born from the bypass machine
to taunt this new person?
Whose image looks back
from my mirror?

Which one of me lies awake to worry
that this pain is IT? Which one says,
I didn't come back from the dead
to take crap from anybody?

Which one?
There just seem to be two,
more Gemini than ever,
talking back to the world,
neither one even trying
to be polite.

I am convinced that statins are the source of my problems that a great deal of time, trouble, discomfort, worry, and money spent by Medicare could have been saved if I had stopped the statins on January 1st for 30 days. After 20 more days without statins, I recorded the following in my diary.

"As of today I am able to 1) double my evening walk, 2) plant flowers with no problems with fatigue, 3) wash windows without aches and pains, 4) do my full exercise routine at the Wellness Center, 5) plan for the Skidmore conference without fear, 6) notice improved eyesight, 7) improved memory, 8) improved digestion, 9) stable weight and 10) enough energy if it is managed carefully."

But here I am at my next cardiology appointment. I announce to the doctor the following, as nicely as I can: "Here is what I am going to do. I am going to assemble my husband and my four children and I am going to tell them, 'You can have me as I am, a lively pain-in-the-neck, but I might drop dead next week without statins, OR I can become the confused, memory-losing zombie at 75 that your great-grandmother Kelly was at 95, if I continue to take statins. You must help me to choose which I will do.' "

Needless to say, my cardiologist was upset. "It doesn't have to be either/or. We can try other things." And so we have. She continues to work with me, aggravation that I am, right up to the present day. Not taking statins does not mean that I can ignore the need to keep my cholesterol in check by some other means. We tried various remedies and ruled out niacin and red yeast rice.

In February, 2013 came vindication of my concerns, as well as more reason to approach these drugs only with careful consultation with one's individual doctor. The FDA has issued a health alert requiring that statins carry labels warning of confusion, memory loss, muscle weakness, and elevated blood sugar leading to Type 2 diabetes.

In "Warning on Statins: FDA more open about risks" by Robert Bazell, chief Science and Health Correspondent for NBC News, (2/29/2013), quotes Dr. Garret Fitzgerald, Chairman of Pharmacology at the University of Pennsylvania, who states, "These warnings should put an end to all the silliness about giving these drugs to everyone."

Everyone from my cardiac surgeon to the FDA agrees that statins can save lives; but they should be used only with clear knowledge that there are risks involved. However, with these new warnings, no longer will patients be told that they are just getting older, forgetful, or even worse, misdiagnosed with Alzheimer's disease

It is interesting to note that the Women's Health Initiative (the massive government study which unearthed the risks and dangers of hormone therapy) comes into play here. A survey of 150,000 women who participated in that study revealed that the older women who took statins were 48% more likely to develop type 2 diabetes. With millions of women being urged to take statins, that is a lot of women who may be innocently damaging their own health.

As I said at the beginning of this lengthy section, I am not a medical authority, and **what I have related should not be used for diagnostic purposes by another patient**. It is a cautionary tale, which you should use to ask questions of your own medical advisors.

I headed off to Skidmore and had a great time. I traveled alone by train and bus without any problems. But I knew full well that I must now learn all that I could about everything I could possibly use to optimize my own physical, emotional, mental and spiritual healing.

To my great surprise, a lecture about women and heart health by a local cardiologist directed me back to Dr. Cohen's view of small doses in a very powerful way. Dr. Steven Guidera, MD is the Director of the Catheterization Lab at the Heart Institute of Doylestown Hospital in Doylestown, PA. When asked what he does about patients who can't take statins because of the side effects, he replied that he uses the very small dose method. "Most people can tolerate statins, the trick is to get the right statin at a dose they can tolerate."

Dr. Guidera said that he gives the patient 5mg of a statin on Mondays—and that is all, for one month. This is a far cry from the 20 to 40 mg per day, doses which many doctors prescribe. If that is OK, he gives another 5mg on Fridays, two doses for another month. "Then we see if we can get them to 5mg three times a week." So far it seems to work, just as Dr. Cohen reported. You can get results without side effects by realizing that only small doses of these very powerful drugs are needed.

So it was off to discuss this with my cardiologist, and see if she would agree to let me try it. After some extended discussion, Dr. Sangrigoli agreed to let me try Dr. Guidera's plan and take 5mg of Simvastatin for one month, then twice a week, then three times a week. This was as long as I continued to take small doses of Losartin (to keep my arteries flexible) and Zetia, (a vegetable compound for lowering cholesterol).

The result—my LDL bottomed out at 85. I have followed this regimen, with supplements COQ 10, with good results. I am able to exercise, garden, do housework and travel without problems as long as I regulate my sleep and use of energy. Who knows? My battle with the statins may yet end in a truce.

Once again, this is MY experience; I relate it only to suggest questions the reader might want to ask of her own physicians.

6

NOBODY TOLD ME ABOUT CORTISOL

Cortisol...the word came up in my reading and I had no idea what it implied. I couldn't help asking if there might really be something wrong with me. As with many other ideas on my long journey, I came upon this one by accident, in an article in the catalogue for the Kripalu Center for Yoga and Health, titled "The Cutting Edge of Trauma Treatment: Healing Through the Body" by Nora Isaacs (Summer, 2009, Kripalu Center for Yoga and Health. Cited with permission)

"Big T" Trauma

Here I discovered that a life-threatening medical procedure (open heart surgery) is classed as "Big T Trauma" by experts in the field of post-traumatic stress. Dr. Bessel van der Kolk is a pioneer in this field and founder of The Trauma Center in Brookline, MA.

As a threat to bodily integrity, according to van der Kolk, "Trauma is a condition under which your body continues to get triggered into believing in an old situation as if you were back there again."

His view was echoed by trauma specialist Dana Moore of the Trauma Center Professional Training Institute. "Often the result of Big T trauma is that a person lives in a hyper-aware, hyper-sensitive state to ensure that the intense life-threatening experience (war, plane crash, earthquake, mugging, rape, massive surgery) doesn't happen again." During a traumatic experience, scientific studies have shown that the body—in the case of my surgery, an unconscious body—undergoes profound chemical changes as the ancient 'fight or flight' reaction kicks in, flooding the body with cortisol and adrenaline to ensure survival."

Among other effects, we now know that the speech center of the brain can shut down and information processing can be affected. Remember that I could not write for six months after my surgery. For me at least, this new information about hyper-arousal would explain the fear and anxiety reactions.

So I wasn't going crazy. Deep within, down on cellular level, my body was still frightened that the surgery would happen again. The least thought/sign of possible danger would set off the alarms sending cascades if survival substances through body and mind. For a long while, more than a year, every situation would be inspected for possible threats: hence the fear-based reaction to everyday events.

However, according to van der Kolk, the answers do not lie in the mental state as much as they do in the body, or the somatic realm. "...Feeling that someone understands your suffering (support groups) is enormously comforting..." *but it doesn't make your body know you are safe. The real method is resetting your physiology."* (Italics mine).

This, of course, means some way of moving that body and he strongly recommends yoga. "It can rewire your brain stem, and change the fear system in your brain." He further states, "To feel what you feel and know what you know *in your body*, can go a long way toward healing." [11] So my regular routine of chair yoga was the right way to go, as was regular massage, and my full exercise routine at Cardiac Rehab.

After The Kripalu Article

I began to research trauma. Attending a lecture by psychologist Dr. Lana Liberto called "Attitude Counts," I began to wonder if I might be suffering from what is called Post Traumatic Stress Syndrome/Disorder (PTSD). After all, my body had suffered a tremendous trauma and all the way down to cellular level, it had no way of knowing the difference between a roadside bomb in Iraq; a plane crash in the Hudson River; an earthquake in China, or seven hours of open heart surgery. The body has been attacked, fought to survive and is deeply afraid that it will happen again; it must therefore stay on the alert.

But nobody told me about cortisol, the big stress hormone, part of our evolutionary protection from danger. It rearranges the body chemistry to ensure survival by sending extra supplies to muscles for flight, and shutting down functions like digestion, which is not needed. As such, it can supply the needed energy to fight back, run away or generally save ourselves from a threat to our well-being. The problem arises when as stated above, the body continues to be alert for trauma that will not be coming, long after the event is over.

Psychologist Neil Fiore, PhD, explains it this way in *New Choices in Natural Healing*. "Consistently evoking the stress response with images of danger in the past, or stress in the future, is tantamount to setting off a false fire alarm in your body."[12]

Cortisol And Stress

In my searching through books on healing modalities, I began reading Belleruth Naparstek's, *Everyday Heroes: Survivors of Trauma and How They Heal*. Initially, I was turned off by the descriptions of other people's traumas–wars, rapes, car accidents, child abuse; they were not like surgery, which is designed to save, not to damage. Instinctively I knew that reading these depressing stories would only add to my own on-and-off bouts of depression.

Early in the book I had found, "One flamboyantly observable biological marker is cortisol, one of the more easily measured hormones that surge through a body triggered by stress." Stress? Heart surgery, cataract surgery which disrupted my vision; diverticulitis; my mother's hip surgery; a colon resection and recovery; my mother's death; and statin problems. Stress—I guess!

In the discussion between the troubling case histories I began to find sections and phrases describing familiar experiences:

The What Ifs scenarios. Getting in the car and wondering if I would have an accident would lead, because I am an imaginative writer, to mentally enacting a whole scenario, all the way through to disaster—and I now realized, to raised blood pressure and general anxiety.

Negative interpretation of ordinary events. Naparstek describes it as, "The bias toward noticing what is worrisome and frightening at the expense of registering what is beautiful and nourishing."[13] I remembered my banging the steering wheel; my daughter scolding me.

Negative and troublesome dreams: Not really nightmares as such, but unpleasant enough, and regular enough to make me not want to go to sleep.

Feeling flat, dead and numb: Getting through a day without caring about anything, without any interest in events around me. Or waking up worried and anxious and not knowing why.

Finally, there was a statement about "feeling unpleasantly stoned," which made me pause. "Indeed these people are stoned—on the endogenous opoids flooding their systems from a disregulated endocrine system."[14]

Say what?

I was beginning to understand a deeper interpretation of the well-known idea that we have a built-in fight or flight system in the most primitive parts of our brains; which is what has allowed mankind to survive for so long. It enables our brains to direct our bodies to enhance certain systems with floods of hormones, in specific combinations, to allow a person to sense and/or escape from danger.

Once the danger has passed, the system is designed to return to proper balance. Indeed other mammals have a high ability to literally "shake off" the hormone flood and return to normal. Rabbits and deer can do it many times a day as they go about their lives evading danger, with no ill effects. But with all of the levels of our human consciousness, from the highest analytical functions to the basest primitive brain sections, humans do not walk away from a major trauma that easily.

So as Naparstek explained, "Our hard-won survival imperative has geared our brains to unquestioningly and automatically remember and deeply imprint any danger related information. All it takes is one terrifying, life-threatening event (seven hours of open heart surgery?) to make a profoundly memorable event."[15] Once this has happened, our major center for processing emotion and sensation, the amygdala, can remain sensitive to the least sign of perceived danger, no matter what the source.

How Cortisol Affects The Body

The concept of body-memory has always been very real to me. I can remember as a kid, after a day of roller skating on city sidewalks, lying in bed and feeling my feet clamped into the skates, the vibrations of the wheels as I fell asleep. Later in life, after surgery for a hysterectomy, my body remembered being moved off the operating table, onto a gurney, and then into my bed.

Even more disconcerting was foot surgery several years later. As I drifted to sleep, I could feel my foot being pressed into the plate to hold it still so a hole could be drilled to place a pin in my toe. Body then "remembered" the whole experience, but there was no pain. In that way I understood what happens when you are anesthetized. Pain centers are shut off, as well as consciousness, but there is no way that the affected cells do not retain some memory of what was done to them. Apply this to open heart surgery, and it is easy to see why traumatic symptoms of whatever nature persist over long periods of time—and why patients are entitled to know about them.

As usual, Dr. Mehmet Oz had a more whimsical explanation, in *YOU Staying Young*, but it did help to clarify what happens when it takes weeks, months or even longer, for the shock to the body to come to terms with all the chemical imbalances triggered by the initial trauma. Each time your body-memory perceives a threat, it happens all over again.

Here is Doctor Oz on what happens in a, "hormonal system that sounds like a Star Wars galaxy: the hypothalamic-pituitary-adrenal (HPA) axis. The stress hormones cycle among these three glands in a feedback loop. When you are faced with a stressor (or a reliving of a stressor, or even suspecting a stressor) the hypothalamus releases CRH, which does a hula dance on your pituitary gland, stimulating it to release another hormone called ACTH into your bloodstream. ACTH then signals your adrenal gland to produce cortisol and adrenaline. Stress over, the cortisol is supposed to cycle back to the hypothalamus and stop the production of CRH." [16]

Researchers have found that the section of the brain charged with quieting down the system after the perceived threat (by now only a memory, relived because of a trigger) has passed, fails to go into gear. The more this is repeated, the more chronic it can become. The result is a state of hypervigilance, chemical imbalance, and mental, emotional and physical symptoms. So there are good reasons for the What Ifs, the negativity, the depression, the anxiety. The trauma has caused observable physiological and hormonal-regulating changes to a greater or lesser degree in the traumatized brain. And the culprit appears to be cortisol.

I had long maintained that my conscious mind does not remember the surgery in the same way as, say a plane crash survivor would, with flashbacks, fear of flying, etc.

However, researchers have found that the same brain changes occurred when a subject was *read* a detailed narrative of her trauma. In my case, repeated readings of the surgeon's notes created a kind of memory. I did this at first out of curiosity, and then repeatedly in preparing certain sections of this book, as well as in the poetry readings I do.

Naparstek calls this, "a condition deliberately designed to elicit flashbacks and to activate the whole biochemical, neurological and emotional cascade."[17]

I was unaware that I was adding to my stress by reading the surgeon's notes. It also explains why I feel a certain discomfort each time I do a public reading of the poems. However, I have learned to work on not allowing the What Ifs to become fully imagined stress-provoking scenarios. I made good progress in breaking what I had considered to be a "habit."

Imagine my surprise to find that it could be, "...first and foremost a matter of unconscious neurophysiological conditioning, rooted in the biochemistry of the traumatized brain. People are unknowingly addicted to their own biochemicals and are thus provoking doses of their own stress neuro-hormones."[18]

How can this be? Me? Addicted? After the adrenaline rush of the stress, comes the endorphin (the feel-good hormone) rush for release. *Both are opoids and both are addictive.* This all goes on beneath any conscious awareness, so how is one to deal with it? Here is where the major theme of this book comes into play. The healing modalities I have used are known to generate endorphins, and thus can put the brakes on the uncontrolled release of the HPA cycle! And patients are entitled to know about them.

According to Elizabeth Scott, MS (In "How Cortisol Affects Your Body' About.com 11/14/2011) higher and prolonged levels of cortisol in the body caused by chronic stress, or the hyper-vigilant state resulting from trauma, can impair your cognitive function, suppress your thyroid, affect muscle tissue, blood sugar, bone density, blood pressure and immune response. Only recently, the notorious belly fat has been added to the list. When I asked Psychologist Dr. Lana Liberto which came first, the cortisol or the belly fat, she replied that the evidence shows that the cortisol comes first.

Scott lists the following as methods for keeping the stress hormones, particularly cortisol, in balance: guided imagery, journaling, exercise, yoga, music, breathing exercises, and sex. Dr. Oz joins in with recommending exercise and sex as the two key stress fighters in his AARP Magazine column. Naparstek suggests the substitution of one endorphin high for another–using imagery, meditation, yoga or exercise. In reminding myself to cut off the scenarios of disaster and create a positive image to contemplate, I was doing this all along, without knowing it!

Of crucial importance for this book is a final quote from Naparstek which describes my relief at learning about and understanding what was happening to me and how I could make progress in dealing with it. She points out that most people get over these uncomfortable symptoms in a few weeks or months. In my case it has taken years, because I was, if not re-traumatized, at least re-stressed due to further surgery and life events.

BUT, she says "For these people (*people like me*) just knowing something about their temporary symptoms and why they occur is valuable and reassuring. [19] (Italics mine) And stress-reducing? And better than prescribing tranquilizers? Education, education, education…

It seems that the research is only beginning to discover all the ways in which the hormones secreted by the HPA cycle, especially cortisol, interact with multiple systems of both mind and body, both dramatically and with great subtlety, possibly over long periods of time. I am still trying to understand why doctors do not educate surgery patients to be aware that if they experience the effects of their disturbed cortisol levels, they "come with the territory;" can be dealt with without medications, and will subside over time.

I only know that I have developed a mantra for when the nameless anxiety sweeps over me, triggered by who-knows-what; or when a day of depressive thinking looms first thing in the morning. I fold my hands over my rebuilt heart and repeat, "It is just the cortisol. It is chemical. It will pass." Finally, over this past year, I use it less and less.

Now surgery, especially the massive "salvage surgery" which I and others have experienced, differs from all the other traumas associated with PTSD symptoms in an important way. All the others are either natural disasters, mechanical failures, actions taken by sick or malevolent persons or wars.

Surgery, as Dr. Oz has said, is "controlled trauma"—horrendous things done to another human being, but with the purpose of saving that person's life: slicing open the chest, bone-sawing the sternum, actually handling the heart, harvesting leg veins for a bypass. In my case, seven hours of inflicting actions on another person which, if done by a maniac, would rival the "Tennessee Chainsaw Massacre."

However, it is more and more recognized that surgery is LIKE all the other traumas in important ways. Even though the patient's conscious mind is non-functional, the deeper survival recesses of the brain activate the same rush of incredibly complex chemical cascades as any other trauma experienced while awake.

This is certainly not to say that these horrendous things should not be done. The incredible surgical skill with which they were carried out saved my life. But it needs to be acknowledged they were horrendous, and that there may be some long-term effects to be dealt with.

PTSD, Deep Trauma And The Poems

It is interesting to see the ideas about PTSD and the deepest levels of cellular reaction to the controlled trauma of surgery reflected in the poems. More interesting is that the poems came before I was ready to write a book, but only after six months separated me from the trauma. For instance, the anger can be seen in "The Sound of Knives." The deep, deep level on which a procedure of this kind is experienced is evident in "The Decider." The almost out-of-body which some patients have is on display in "The Gospel According to Intensive Care." Living with the scary is portrayed in "The Calf," and "The Revenant." My year-long struggle to resolve the statin situation resulted in the lament of "To Gaia."

Education, Education, Education

The patient is entitled to be educated about what is going on, and to be offered sympathetic and humane contact and support from people who have "been there, done that" as well as medical professionals. The patient is also entitled to be made aware of the many healing modalities of integrative medicine which may help them to recover. So often they are offered only pills.

Case in point: In a hospital pamphlet, the possibility of emotional issues is acknowledged sympathetically. The patient is advised to seek out a physician, counselor, family member, clergyman, or in the extreme, a psychologist or psychotherapist. No mention is made of support from other heart patients, or any of the now research-based healing modalities that are readily available in most communities.

The scene, my cardiac rehab facility: A new member is adjusting to life after 12 weeks of hospital rehab and he is scared. "Every little pain—you think, is it serious? Should I call the doctor? My wife doesn't understand."

"Of course," I reply. "She has never had heart surgery. That is what you can get from the folks here. We've been there, done that, and we can sympathize."

Another woman chimes in with what could be our mantra "You live with the scary."

Being alone with your fears generates stress and that can lead to anxiety and depression. But you can learn to judge your symptoms and to manage your fears. Support is crucial. Education about what is happening to you is crucial. Every patient is not equipped to make the effort that I have made in preparing this manuscript.

Psychologist Lana Liberto specializes in recovery from trauma of various kinds. She says, "I believe that every heart surgery patient should, as an integrative part of their medical treatment, have a consultation with a psychologist. This is not because they are crazy, but to give them permission to feel what they feel—depression, anxiety, anger—as a normal part of recovery." (Interview, 8/20/2015)

Doctors and hospitals can go a long way toward gently educating post-surgery patients about what can be happening to their bodies, minds and spirits. But this can take place only if doctors and hospitals themselves are educated in the value of using integrative medicine's evidence-based modalities combined with conventional treatments. My education came from my own experience and my own research. I will try to share both with the reader in the rest of this book .

PART II

A BEGINNING

> *"The human body is the physician of its own illness."*
> Hippocrates

7

THE DIFFERENCE BETWEEN HEALING AND CURING

So what did I learn from my body, and with my mind, to heal both of them and my spirit in these long and life-giving wonderful years? Let us begin with some definitions from the *Oxford English Dictionary.* Then we will hear from Michael Lerner, McArthur Fellow, founder of Commonweal, and on staff at the Medical School of UC San Francisco; from Mischala Joy Devi in *The Healing Path of Yoga*; from Norman Cousins in *The Healing Heart;* from Caroline Myss, a pioneer in energy medicine, and from Penelope Quest, Canadian author of *Self-Healing with Reiki.*

Here is what the dictionary says, along with my comments in italics:

Repair: The action or process of restoring something to unimpaired condition by replacing or fixing worn or damaged parts. *Well that fits. They replaced my mitral valve, repaired my tricuspid valve, and repaired my clogged/damaged arteries with parts salvaged from my left leg.*

Rehabilitate: To restore a person to some degree of normal life by training after an illness or injury. *Restoring to 'some degree' is what Cardiac Rehab will do for the rest of my life, as long as I keep showing up.*

Recover: To regain health, strength, or consciousness; to get well. *Health? Back to some degree. Strength? I keep working on it.*

Consciousness? I know a lot more now about how various systems interact within my body, physically, chemically, emotionally, etc. Get well? Not really an end-point, but an ongoing process of living, of being well.

Cure: Successful medical treatment; the action or process of healing a sick person, or a thing that does this—to treat surgically or medically to restore health—to relieve of illness. *My medical procedures have been quite successful from an allopathic (mainstream) point of view. My heart (and eyes and colon) have been restored to health. My heart disease illness, has of course, not been relieved, or ever will be. No doctor said to me at my five-year anniversary that I was free of heart disease.*

Heal: To become whole or sound again. In mind, body and spirit. The *Oxford English Dictionary* uses heal to define cure. *But in modern times, with so much of conventional medicine involving mechanical procedures rather than concern for the mind, body, spirit, heal and cure are no longer the same thing. It is one of the major concepts I had to learn. Cure comes from the outside. Heal is what you do for yourself.*

Bill Moyers' *Healing and the Mind*, Michael Lerner agrees: "Curing is the scientific effort to change what is happening in the body. [20] Curing is what allopathic mainstream medicine has to offer, when it can, and what the physician brings to you." [21]

It cannot be said enough times, that this is what kept me from dying; the medical miracles for which I will always be grateful. However, as Lerner and so many others point out, and I have spent years learning, it is not the whole story.

"Healing is what you bring to the encounter with your (disease/problem) and with mainstream medicine. Healing comes from inner resources. It is the human experience of the effort to recover." [22]

It is the subject of this book! Lerner further states:

"We need to bring the old wisdom together with mainstream medicine so that main-stream medicine can become more humane and compassionate in the application of its technologies." [23]

This is not to say that I myself was ever treated in a way that could be defined as not humane. It is that in so many situations, mainstream medicine seems to think that repair and cure are sufficient to complete the healing process. They are not.

Norman Cousins, in his best-selling *The Healing Heart*, says it this way: "A physician should be able to mobilize and release all those forces in a human being that work for regeneration and repair." [24] Or at least be able to point the patient to someone who can do that, like the healers of the integrative medical modalities. The skills to do these things should be being taught in our medical schools.

In her comprehensive work, *The Healing Path of Yoga*, Mischala Joy Devi reminds us on page 1, "While stressful events around us may not change, we can LEARN how to respond skillfully to life's difficulties." On page 5, she states it quite plainly, in one of the best statements I have seen:

"We are the healers. Taking responsibility for our own health and well-being, our bodies and minds reveal the secrets of balance, harmony, and the release of energy for healing. This decreases the need for someone else to FIX us. We learn more about our bodies than anyone else. We then consult with professionals as partners in our own healing process, not as FIXERS." [25]

Caroline Myss, author of the best-selling *Anatomy of the Spirit: The Seven Stages of Power and Healing*, says it this way:

"The process of curing is passive; that is, the patient is inclined to give over his or her authority to the physician and to prescribed treatments…so that responsibility for healing lies with the doctor. The chemical treatments of conventional medicine require no conscious participation on the part of the patient. Healing, on the other hand, is an active internal process…In holistic therapies the patient's willingness to participate fully in his own healing is necessary for success." [26]

Finally, in *Self-Healing with Reiki*, Penelope Quest, British author and Reiki Master, distinguishes four areas of healing:

Physical Healing: Might mean eradicating the illness, or improving symptoms while you work on other aspects. *(Applies to me because I will never be free of the conditions of my rebuilt heart, although the use of integrative modalities works toward helping me to heal)*

Emotional Healing: Includes calming fears (a large and ongoing job for me) accepting limitations (4another big job) and letting go of anger or resentment. (*I have enough to do with the first two; I have not had much here.)*

Mental/Psychological Healing: Allowing you to think differently about your illness, or helping to let go of negative attitudes.*(Possibly in terms of realizing that you are not as limited as you may think)*

Spiritual Healing: Helps you to develop a more loving and forgiving relationship with yourself, and allows for greater self-expression and creativity. It can also help to create a peaceful transition for those facing death. (*Learning to love yourself is mentioned prominently in virtually every source I consulted. Lack of self-esteem really prevents healing.)*

In the long haul of recovery and healing I figured things out for myself by listening to what my body told me, and then found it validated in research both in conventional and integrative medicine. The kinds of things I learned convinced me that while the miracles of modern medicine can repair our failing and damaged bodies, only the individual can heal the body, the mind and the spirit. The key to that healing is, among other things, knowledge of what has happened and is happening to the entity known as YOU.

It has taken me more than five years to even begin to realize the process of learning about my body, mind and spirit. It took lots of reading, asking questions of doctors and health practitioners; even more experiencing and experimenting, but I continue to teach myself what I need to know. It is this above all: Mind, body, and spirit are linked in very real physiological, chemical and spiritual ways, and all three must be integrated for true healing to take place.

The more I thought about it over the long months when I felt almost constantly ill at ease, vaguely threatened, the more it seemed as though I had been through some awful disaster, even if it did save my life. I was unconscious, whatever that is, while all this was being done to me so I did not have an intellectual framework for the cracking open of my bones, the handling of my heart, the bypass machine. According to the surgeon's notes, my heart did not respond to stimulation at first—my body was ready to quit.

And like any other threat to the life force's existence, the body marshals all of the chemical, hormonal, and energy forces to save itself, or it will die. Modern medical science has learned to assist these forces with machines, medications, and careful chemical support, after inflicting the lifesaving "disaster" of the operation. So why isn't that enough? Why isn't "fixing" your heart (a phrase doctors do use) the end of the story? You are conscious when the initial trauma is over, but your mind, body and spirit must come together and come to terms with what that means for the rest of your life.

During the early weeks and months of my recovery I faithfully performed my physical therapy and took my meds. Doctors were sympathetic—even offered me pills. They were seriously concerned about depression and anxiety, especially in the first year after heart surgery. But no one offered me the healing modalities of integrative medicine as ways to manage my healing. I had to figure it out for myself. Many truly caring doctors do not appreciate, even now, the unbreakable link between body, mind and spirit as one system, and do not address these factors with their patients. I will discuss how that could be changed in a later section.

The reader will notice that along with my personal experiences, I am making ample use of the views of medical doctors, PhD researchers and integrative medicine practitioners. This is to validate my insistence that both research studies and medical practices in major institutions have validated these healing modalities.

> *"Illness of any kind, as evidenced by any physical or emotional problems, is simply blocked or stuck energy; chi that has gotten withheld from the general flow, tipping the body/mind out of balance. So any kind of symptom, be it coronary artery disease or ulcers, depression or back spasm, is some form of blocked or separated energy."*
> Bellaruth Naparstek in
> *Staying Well with Guided Imagery*

8

ENERGY, MERIDIANS AND CHAKRAS

Before moving on to my own experiences with the various healing modalities which aided in my recovery, it seems helpful to discuss the over-arching ideas on which many of them are based. The exact nature of what is referred to as Chi or qi for centuries is not yet known. However, modern science works constantly toward an answer. Dr. Oz, in *YOU Staying Young*, agrees. "It's these energy fields—your life force, your chi, your intangible aura–that we believe will be the next great frontier in medicine."[27]

According to principals of ancient medical practice which are several thousand years old, energy moves through the body along specific lines called meridians. Detailed charts of these meridians form the basis of practices in acupuncture, reflexology, Tai Chi others. Along the spinal column these energy forces form vortexes at specific locations called chakras. There are believed to be seven of them from the bottom of the spine (the coccyx) to the top of the head.

The four-thousand years old "Yellow Emperor's Classic of Internal Medicine" first articulated these ideas. Over the next two thousand years, Chinese doctors discovered a system of channels and points on the body that if correctly touched and or stimulated, could relieve pain and speed healing. One author has suggested thinking of meridians as a subway system with fourteen main lines and three-hundred and sixty five stops.

Rarely practicing surgery, the ancient Chinese believed that illness was the result of imbalances in the flow of these forces. The imbalances could be caused by unhealthy living, injury, or imbalances coming from outside forces in nature. Moderation in all things was, and still is, the guiding principle.

Fast forward to the present and one still finds these principles at work in healing practices. In many cases, these are now able to be measured with sophisticated electronic devices, and studied in controlled experiments. One reason for the persistence of skepticism about these ideas is that the validating information is scattered among numbers of obscure but reputable journals in narrow fields of interest. The fact remains that the information is there, for anyone who takes the time and trouble to look at it.

Energy healer Anodea Judith, in *Eastern Body, Western Mind* says, "The inner and outer realms are NOT separate, but we lack a system for tying them together." [28] She, along with many others in the field, use the ancient concept of chakras to suggest a possible system for accomplishing this. Their studies range from ancient wisdom to the cutting edge of contemporary biochemistry and neurology.

Judith explains it this way. "A chakra is a center of organization that receives, assimilates, and expresses life force energy. It refers to a spinning sphere of bioenergetics activity emanating from the major nerve ganglia branching forward from the spinal column." [29]

Dr. Memet Oz relates, in *Healing from the Heart* "Practitioners believe that energy flows within the body through channels called meridians, with seven major energy centers called chakras (The Sanskrit word for wheel) aligned along the spine. Each chakra emits and absorbs a different life force (The Chinese call it chi or qi) and it governs different areas, even organs, in the body." [30]

Caroline Myss, PhD, recognized as a pioneer in energy medicine, in *Anatomy of the Spirit* explains, "Eastern cultures teach that the human body contains seven energy centers...chakras are vertically aligned running from the base of the spine to the crown of the head." [31] Positive and negative experiences register a memory in cell tissue as well as in the energy field.

As neurobiologist Dr. Candace Pert, PhD has proven, neuropeptides— the chemicals triggered by our emotions—are thoughts converted into matter. Our emotions reside physically in our bodies and interact with our cells and tissues." [32] "In this way, your biography—that is, the experiences that make up your life—becomes your biology." [33]

It is the late Candace Pert whose groundbreaking work in neurobiology

73

and scientific credentials allowed her to speak with authority regarding the concept of energy healing and the chakra system. She did so in her best known work, *Molecules of Emotion,* and more informally in a CD called *Healing the Hurting, Shining the Light.* (2009, Candace Pert, Magic Bullets, LLC) where she says, "Ancient peoples imagined spinning wheels of different colors, at different levels of our body. We now recognize this as the spinal column with branches of nerves connected to all parts of the body."

In her CD she explains that we are only aware of a tiny piece of what goes on in our body/mind. "There is no difference. The same molecules run digestion, breathing, immunity, feelings, even memories and belief systems...Our cells are constantly being born, moving, dying, being replaced—even our brain is renewed by cells born deep in our bones...Numerous types of information molecules called neuropeptides are concentrated at various locations along the neuroaxis...Interestingly, these nodal points tend to correspond with the sites of the chakras...Each node is a module which processes information, alters its ebb and flow, up and down the body, regulates physiology, and colors mood and perception."

With credentials including a pharmacology degree from Johns Hopkins University, a post as Chief of Section on Brain Biochemistry at the National Institutes of Mental Health, Professor of Physiology and Biochemistry at Georgetown University and private research in her own laboratory, Pert spoke with Bill Moyers for his *Healing the Mind.* "Intelligence is in every cell of your body. It is not confined to the space above your neck." [34] In order to understand all of this someday, Pert believes, "We're going to have to bring in that extra-energy realm, the realm of spirit and soul that Descartes kicked out of Western thought." [35]

Gleaned from Pert and Judith, the following is a brief chart of the chakra system. Each chakra is associated with parts of the body, an aspect of our identity, and a color based on its vibration. These develop from the bottom up and are associated with various stages of our growth toward spiritual and physical maturity. Energy, however you call it (chi, ki, prana, mana) runs the whole thing.

First chakra: base of spine; "root" chakra; physical identity—"I feel grounded"—self-preservation; color is red, slowest vibration of visible light.

Second: lower abdomen; emotional identity—"I feel nurtured"—sexuality; gratification; color is orange.

Third: solar plexis/diaphragm; ego identity—"I feel powerful"—self-esteem; self definition; color is yellow.

Fourth: Heart; social identity—"I give and receive love"—harmony; self-acceptance; color is green.

Fifth: Throat—creative identity—"I express myself and take action"—self-expression; color is sky blue.

Sixth: Brow/third eye; archetypal identity—"What I imagine comes true"—intuition; self-reflection; color is indigo.

Seventh: crown of head; universal identity—"I am sending and receiving electro-magnetic energy from the universe"—self-knowledge; color is violet (highest vibration of visible light)/or pearly white (union of all colors).

According to Pert, science tells us that there are more neuronal connections to the brain in the crown chakra than anywhere else. It also tells that the heart contains every peptide neuronal substance ever measured, that the heart does not really beat steadily, but shifts and regulates the electrical energy of the whole body. All these beliefs correspond to the placement of the chakras by the ancient beliefs.

As explained by Judith, loss of any of these identities will block that chakra, and such blockages can lodge in our musculature and effect breathing, metabolism, and emotional states. This in turn manifests in relationships, work, creativity and even belief systems. Dr. Oz comments, "Removing blockages of the life force along the meridians, creating balance and dispelling illness is the goal of all energy healers."[36]

How is this done? Recognizing the block and the associated chakra is essential. Then applying exercises and techniques to achieve a balance of energy forces. Judith includes the following: body work, meditation, discussion groups, imaging, sound therapy, exercise, and surprisingly, real-world tasks.[37] For me gardening, cleaning house, or taking a walk have proven useful in restoring balance, in addition to the more formal actions which are detailed in the rest of this book.

That energy fields move through, and around the human body, uniting mind and body chemically, neurologically, physically, emotionally and even spiritually, is no longer to be dismissed. Even the *Readers Digest Family Guide to Natural Medicine* agrees, "Recent research in the field of psychoneuroimmunology (PNI) has shown that the brain, endocrine and immune systems are interconnected by a series of neural pathways. (Those ancient Chinese were on to something). These pathways may form a communications network that enables mind and body to influence each other."[38]

There is the modern practice of acupressure or shiatsu, where pressure is applied at specific meridians where centuries of experience indicate that balance can be returned. For headache relief, press the web of flesh between thumb and forefinger. To relieve nausea, press the thumb into an area two inches above the crease in the wrist.

Acupuncture, another ancient technique, is believed to have originated using hands also, only later developing into the use of needles. The tiny needles are believed to stimulate the meridians and increase healing energy flow. While awaiting surgery for diverticulitis, acupuncture needles in my abdomen (painless) relieved the pain in that area.

Reflexology, or massage of hands or feet, works on the same principle. Detailed charts indicate points which connect, by way of meridians, to specific points, joints and organs. For instance the place where the big toe connects to the foot is connected to the neck. A spot in the center of the arch on the bottom of the foot connects to the kidneys. These systems can be used for both discovery and healing; pain when a particular spot is pressed can indicate a physical problem. Reiki is based on the idea that properly attuned, simply laying on of the hands can transfer balance and healing energy. Various types of massage have their origins in these theories.

Once attuned to the energy flow in your body by using these modalities, the chakra system makes wonderful sense. Meanwhile, I have found healing relief in my sampling of these modalities with reputable practitioners, as well as rethinking my approach to two everyday realities: sleep and food.

> *"More important than knowing what disease a patient has, is knowing what patient has the disease."*
>
> William Osler,
> The Father of Modern Medicine

9

INTEGRATIVE MEDICINE

What is happening with these forms of relieving suffering, which are called by a variety of names–comprehensive, alternative, integrative medicine? Some practitioners and authors use the CAM acronym. I prefer the single term integrative, because it implies most strongly the union of all forms of healing, both conventional and nonconventional.

"Alternative" implies that these methods, some of them thousands of years old, should be employed "instead of" modern medical science. Nothing could be further from the truth. Some of our most advanced conventional medical centers employ these methods as a matter of course, and advance the research into their effectiveness. However, there are far too many on the other side of this unnecessary divide who have yet to be convinced, and to have their knowledge increased. I have written this book to add my voice to the convincers.

As far back as 2006, a PBS documentary called "The New Medicine" presented the views of seven physicians from such centers. (www.pbs.org/thenewmedicine/using_act.html March, 2006).

In discussing the origins of integrative medicine, Dr. Dennis Novack of the Drexel University College of Medicine reminds us that for thousands of years physicians were shamans, healers, priests. He worries that contemporary physicians are so caught up in the technology that they have lost sight of their "priestly" functions. According to Novack, modern physicians need a better sense of the feelings, worries and experience of illness that the patient brings. He concludes, "What we see in the microscope and the lab results is the disease. All the meaning that the patient brings is the illness."

Dr. Brian Berman of the University of Maryland School of Medicine emphasizes that integrative medicine is a much broader concept than complementary or alternative medicine; that they are more specific modalities to be integrated with conventional medicine. He offers an interesting insight from the blending of integrative medicine with conventional care. "It offers self-care for both physician and patient. These experiences of mindfulness allow us to evaluate our own inner life and how we interact with our patients."

In discussing how medicine is changing, Dr. Tanya Edwards of the Cleveland Clinic Foundation says that we have only just begun the process of integration to include teaching and faculty development in medical schools. She strongly advocates, "Breaking down walls, the barriers from a different cultural outlook." Using energy medicine as an example, she admits, 'We don't understand it yet, but if it works, and it seems to, we should be using it. In another fifty years we may understand it."

Closest to my own experience is Dr. Tracey Gaudet of the Duke Center for Integrative Medicine, whose view is that "Conventional medicine is not prepared to fully address the transformation of a patient with a serious illness or surgery in body, mind, spirit, relationships, etc. The health care system seems to say, "You're done, we fixed you; you're finished." But they are not done, Dr. Gaudet asserts. "It's just the beginning; everything has shifted. The crux of the matter is how we can help patients come out on the other side, not disempowered and not whole, but transformed to a whole other level of health." This is the journey my book describes.

A new definition of health beyond the "absence of illness", the one currently in place, is needed, in the opinion of Dr. Richard Davidson of the W.M. Keck Lab for Functional Brain Imaging and Behavior of the University of Wisconsin. He believes that a more positive "presence of health" should be cultivated and concludes, "We have a lot to learn about physical and mental health in coming years as scientists learn more with regard to this definition."

One need look no further than the National Institutes of Health (NIH) for convincing evidence that modern medicine is including these modalities. Part of the NIH is now the National Center for Complementary and Alternative Medicine (NCCAM) which does studies and defines and reviews approaches to health care that are outside the realm of conventional medicine as practiced in the United States.

In the same PBS video, Dr. Margaret Chesney of the NIH outlines the three most important strategies of the NCCAM to offer patients s full array of choices. "We want to give all the choices and tools we can for a good quality of life, and for physical and mental well-being by doing the following: Supporting the science to help us understand what is safe and effective; training people to do this research for the public; and providing authoritative sources to disseminate this information to the public."

According to Lawrence Chilnick in *Heart Disease: The Essential Guide for the Newly Diagnosed*, here is how the NCCAM indicates that the basics of these approaches can be divided:[39]

Whole medical systems based upon complete systems of theory and practice such as Ayurvedic and Chinese medicine from Asia, and homeopathic and naturopathic from the West. I have not made use of these so far.

Mind-Body Medicine recognizes the scientific proof that emotions effect biology, and includes meditation, prayer, mental healing, imaging, support groups, music, laughter and art therapies. I have made successful use of virtually all of these.

Biologically-based Practices include herbs, foods and dietary supplements. I have also used these.

Manipulative and Body-Based Practices are based on moving various parts of the body and include chiropractic, osteopathic manipulation and massage. Here again, I have used these.

Energy Medicine and Biofield Therapies Studies continue to prove the existence of such fields, but they include qi gong, Reiki and therapeutic touch, which I have used. All of these offer ample examples of the much disdained "anecdotal evidence".

Indeed, Noman Cousins, in his book *The Healing Heart: Antidotes to Panic and Helplessness* says, "Individual experiences, especially in cases of recovery or cure are suspect. The adjective used to describe these experiences is 'anecdotal.' Few words in the medical vocabulary carry more connotations of scorn, even contempt, than 'anecdotal.'"[40]

It is interesting to note that among those who have established

Integrative or Complementary medicine facilities within large respected medical complexes, they have come to their beliefs by learning from their patients and from their own personal experiences. Dr. Memet Oz, long before he was a TV personality, (1998) wrote a book called *Healing From the Heart: How Unconventional Wisdom Unleashes the Power of Modern Medicine.* In it he made the case for the Integrative Medicine Group he established at New York Presbyterian Hospital/Columbia University in the 1990s. Here they have done research into topics ranging from the impact of what patients may hear during surgery to attempting to measure the energy from energy healers' hands using Kirlian photography.

Patients are offered massage, imagery, music and affirming tapes before, during, and after surgery, as well as a variety of other healing modalities; they have been doing it for more than fifteen years. Why? "Because," Dr. Oz says, "The reality is that modern medicine does not understand all human diseases and that patients crave an increasing role in solving their own illnesses."[41]

Dr. Mimi Guarneri, founder and CEO of Pacific Pearl, an integrative medicine facility in San Diego, came to the field by a similar route. As a dynamic, old-school allopathic heart surgeon, she gradually realized that there was much more to the heart than plumbing. As her practice evolved because of her experiences with patients, a personal experience cemented her ideas. Seriously ill with a virus she contracted in the OR, she encountered a nurse who was also an energy healer. A hands-on session with this woman cured her and led to a dramatic change in her approach, the founding of the Integrative Medicine Center, and to her book, *The Heart Speaks.*

In the previously mentioned New Medicine video, Dr. Guarneri frankly outlines what she thinks conventional medicine has been missing in recent years. She states that we gave the spirit to the priests, the mind to the psychiatrists and the heart to the cardiologists, and it is time to practice what she calls, "Whole person medicine. Don't chop people up. The goal is getting toward a full life." She laments the loss of the partnership between patients and physicians, describing too much of current practice as "Do as I say, not as I do, and when you fall apart I will fix you."

Dr. Guarneri's preferred approach is "Let's take a look at what we can do as a team. Why do you think you needed that stent I just put in for you?

I am here to be your coach. I will give you the tools, but it has to come from you. You can't say just give me a pill and I can go out and eat pork ribs tonight."

One of my favorite examples of true "integrative" medicine comes from my heart surgeon, Dr. James McClurkin. When I asked him in an interview for an opinion about yoga, he replied that he has used it himself and recommends it highly, especially for cardiac patients. It seems that heart surgeons are prone to back problems from standing in awkward positions for many hours. Yoga exercises alleviated his problem. He further related that as a med student stressed after a difficult day, he used imaging exercises to help him relax and sleep.

Faced with questions about the use of some healing modality, many in the medical professionals ask, "Where is the research? These would be fine, but they need to be evidence-based." The evidence is there. However, it is often scattered through very specific journals or stretched across a number of disciplines, and thus takes major effort to assemble.

A list of books that have been helpful to me in my quest for true healing will be found in the appendix. It is not long, as book lists go, but it contains a wide variety of ideas to be considered as one navigates the healing process. It represents research, studies, quotations and recommendations from literally hundreds of traditional MD's, PhD's and licensed practitioners that verify the usefulness of these modalities. What is most common about the advice they offer? See your doctor; do not medicate without consulting your doctor; check with your doctor before beginning any new therapy.

Indeed Dr. Anthony Komaroff, senior physician at Brigham and Women's Hospital in Boston and editor-in-chief of Harvard Health Publications, in his syndicated column, remarks when discussing pain issues, "I've had patients respond well to chiropractic, manipulation, acupuncture, massage and yoga." But before that he says, "First, call your doctor", and then he recommends a prescription for pain.

In her groundbreaking imagery study, *Invisible Heroes: Survivors of Trauma and How They Heal,* psychologist Belleruth Naperstek presents a long list of conditions, including massive surgery, for which imagery is "research proven" to be effective in healing.[42] It is accompanied by a numbered note. The citation of the research at the back of the book, for this single note, takes up one and one third pages of fine print. It includes everything from the AMA Journal to "Alternative and Complementary Therapies in Health and Medicine."

In her initial book, *Staying Healthy With Guided Imagery*, Naparstek cites at least fourteen medical centers where physicians are reporting the benefits of imagery in a wide variety of situations.[43] There is no lack of research in the field of integrative medicine.

According to Dr. Guarneri in *The Heart Speaks*, "Research has shown that stress reducers such as visualizations (imagery), hypnosis, deep breathing, meditation and yoga have measureable effects on cardiac risk, helping to relax arteries and reduce levels of stress hormones."[44]

Sound therapy, much wider than music, has a long history of validating studies, as do yoga, acupuncture, meditation. Studies which will be quoted in the section on exercise are being carried out at major universities to validate the benefits of keeping active for heart patients and many others. And of course, my own body has provided evidence of this benefit. No matter how lousy I feel when I enter Cardiac Rehab, the pool, or my yoga class, when I leave I feel better. This is all the "evidence" that many of us need. What I was able to teach myself about healing was learned in two ways: my own research and experimenting on my own body. Each one validated the other, as the reader will see.

For patients looking for a way to be part of this new approach to healing, and hoping to find a physician who practices this way, it is now possible for a physician to become board certified in integrative medicine, just as it is in other specialties. Overseen by the American Association of Physician Specialties, Inc. (as are all board certifications) a group of dedicated integrative medicine practitioners have spent almost twenty years defining terms, assembling criteria and designing exams. Beyond the work at major medical centers, any physician who is willing to meet the criteria and pass the exam can now be certified by the American Board of Integrative and Holistic Medicine.

The ABIHM defines integrative medicine as the practice of medicine that:

- reaffirms the relationship between practitioner and patient
- focuses on the whole person
- is informed by evidence

- makes use of all appropriate therapeutic approaches of healthcare professionals and disciplines, to achieve optimal health and healing.

A reader should not assume that the physicians who have accomplished this decades-long work are outside the mainstream of major medical centers offering both allopathic and integrative medicine approaches. They include Mimi Guarneri MD FACC ABHIM, former director of Integrative Medicine Center at Scripps in San Diego, and now of her own facility, Pacific Pearl, in La Jolla,CA; Randy Horowitz, MD PhD, Medical Director of the University of Arizona Center for Integrative Medicine; Roberta Lee, MD Vice Chair of the Department Of Integrative Medicine at Beth Israel in New York; Patrick Hannaway MD, Director of the Center for Functional Medicine at the Cleveland Clinic; Gerard Mullen MD, Associate Professor in the Department Of Medicine at Johns Hopkins University; Scott Shannon MD, Professor of Child and Adolescent Psychiatry at the University of Colorado; Tieroanoma Low Dog MD, Chief Medical Officer of Weil Lifestyles in Phoenix Arizona, and Mikail Kogan, MD, Medical Director of the George Washington University Center for Integrative Medicine.

In a recent video produced by the ABIHM, these practitioners discuss the importance of an integrative medicine approach to health care, how it differs from the mainstream as currently practiced, and why formal certification is essential.

Guarneri reminds us that integrative medicine involves prevention, use of medical traditions from other cultures, concentrating on the underlying causes of disease and teaching patients to care for themselves. Along with several others, Mullen states that patients are actively seeking competent physicians who treat the whole patient, and Kagan adds that in light if this, it is essential that high standards be established.

There are essential differences with mainstream medicine. Horowitz calls it a "bigger black bag" which allows for consideration of lifestyle, diet, activity, mental state—a different way to approach the whole patient. Shannon agrees, pointing out that he uses integrative medicine in his psychiatric practice with good results. Hathaway says simply, that it is the modern-day application of what has always been considered good medicine.

Why is formal certification so important? Mullen explains that it allows physicians to market themselves as practitioners on whom patients can rely, and allows for them to make and maintain contacts with other practitioners on a regular basis through conferences. Horowitz is pleased that this provides a high standard as well as a well thought out level of training in this growing field. Low Dog ends by pointing that the ABIHM is now part of a consortium of over fifty medical schools and health science centers, and that "It is time," for this recognition. For a list of certified integrative medicine specialists, contact the American Board of Integrative and Holistic Medicine at http://www.abpsus.org/integrativemedicine.

The View From Grand View

Once again, there is more to the story than big-deal research centers. I had the pleasure of encountering Grand View Hospital, a mid-size community hospital in Sellersville, Pennsylvania, about 45 miles North of Philadelphia. Mostly suburban, with vestiges of its rural past, its population is comprised of professionals, working people and a few farmers. It is an open caring place, comfortable enough with integrative medicine to stage a conference about it.

"We were stunned," is how their PR person Mary Karpa described the community reaction. "Space was filled weeks before the event; we had to create a waiting list!"

On a sunny Fall morning I was treated to lectures and demonstrations of yoga, massage, Tai Chi and Chi Qong, chiropractic, acupuncture, natural foods and balanced heart health, by doctors and practitioners of healing modalities. All this was presented around Grand View's definition of integrative medicine: "A whole-person approach to medical care."

The keynote speaker, Dr. William Kracht, DO, of the Woodland Healing Research Center, emphasized that the two ideas—that the body has a marvelous ability to heal itself, and that the mind influences healing—go all the way back to Hippocrates. Dr. Rebecca Nice, a family and integrative physician, recommended, "Laughter, meditation, prayer, exercise, massage, doing something you love, and getting enough sleep." Neurologist Roy Jaekel, MD, pointed out that chronic nerve and muscle pain often responds to healing therapies when all else fails to offer relief. With slides and humor, Todd Aldefer, MD encourages patients to understand that exercise is the greatest factor in a long and healthy life.

Demonstrations featured the methods discussed in the lectures. Neil Matthews, MD a family physician, received his acupuncture training at Harvard. His live patient was John Minnich, MD, who wanted to learn more about acupuncture for his orthopedic practice. Between demonstrations, he donned a suit and gave a lecture on building healthier body and bones with integrative medicine.

Beyond a one-time event, this hospital provides a massage therapist, yoga, meditation, and Tai Chi classes, as well as nutrition counseling at the hospital. Doctors are comfortable referring patients who ask, "What more can I do?" to local practitioners of acupuncture and chiropractic. Some staff physicians also have auxiliary practices in healing modalities and there is an active referral network to these sources.

How did all this come about? According to Karpa, "I think it goes back decades, to our physical therapy department. It seems as if it has always been here. We are embracing more and more of it." Planning Director Stephanie Weaver adds, "Several of our staff may have a somewhat different mind-set, but they are respected here as medical providers."

Indeed these practices have always been there, many of them for centuries. Integrative medicine brings these modalities together with 21st Century medicine. As doctors Stephen Sinatra and James C. Roberts say in *Reverse Heart Disease Now: Stop Deadly Cardiovascular Plaque before It's Too Late*, "The future must bring about a union in which there will be no separate alternative medicine or conventional medicine. Instead we must have smart medicine, in which physicians consider combinations of nutrition, lifestyle, pharmacology and surgery to prevent or treat cardiovascular disease. Hopefully, this union will occur in time to help you and your family, and before our expensive disease management approach bankrupts the Medicare and Medicaid programs."[45]

Welcome to the future.

PART III

HEART MENDING

> *"People who sleep fewer than six hours a night have a fifty percent risk of viral infections and an increased risk of heart disease and stroke."*
>
> Dr. Memet Oz in
> *YOU Staying Young*

10

SLEEP

I never knew how much it mattered. My lack of it over many years could explain a lot. I have always been a night owl. My mother often joked that being born at 9:45 PM was the cause. Getting up in the morning has always been a challenge, which I have ascribed to a generally sluggish metabolism. Caught between these two characteristics, for many years I simply did without.

In college, when the challenging courses, papers due, "all-nighters," commuting to campus, and working on the college paper, took their toll, my body would respond in a way that I understand now, but didn't then. When my physical being had had enough, I would be laid low with a high fever. Nothing else, but the temperature would keep me in bed for several days, until I had rested sufficiently to return to school.

Being a stay-at-home mom for fourteen years raising four closely spaced children only cemented my nighttime habits. It was always easier to do some things when my "helpers" were asleep. To this day, I bake Christmas cookies at night. The year I was home on sabbatical writing *Gifted Grownups*, it took me many weeks to adjust myself to writing in the daytime.

"I'll sleep when I'm dead," was my mantra in the years when a house, a husband, four teenagers, a full-time job teaching Advanced Placement English, and graduate school meant that four to five hours of sleep was what I had with which to get through my life. I actually believed those who said that sleep was highly overrated. I know better now, and I often wonder if the slow subtle damage to my heart began a long time ago. A number of recent studies have verified the claim that those who sleep less than six hours on a regular basis do not live as long.

One summer I tried an experiment. Taking advantage of the go-to-bed-when-you-please and wake-up-when-you-please of summer break, I kept track of how long I usually slept. It turned out to be between 8 and 9 hours. Of course once school started I went right back to my old bad habits, sometimes catching up on weekends. Current research now tells us that is not possible. A pattern, much more subtle than the college one, was present.

I would plow through my workaholic lifestyle—which I didn't recognize as workaholic; I just did what I had to do. But every year, in late February or early March, I would have a flu type illness that would send me to bed and keep me out of work for a week. I learned to husband my sick days to provide for it. Then it would be back to the same stressful pace of teaching, grad school, kids, house, husband, and increasingly, taking care of my elderly mother, a 40-minute drive away in New Jersey.

One small episode of common sense occurred in the last year before my retirement from teaching, a bit late in the game. My office and classes were at one end of our block-long high school, and the cafeteria at the other. Lunch was usually crammed between helping kids who appeared at my door just as I was heading out. I was incapable of saying no, so I'd grab a yoghurt and gulp it down in the five minutes I had left for myself. Or walking the length of the building with my lunch, I'd eat my daily soft pretzel to save time for paper grading and planning.

One day I mused as I walked along, *If I ate my sandwich too, I'd have time to work all through lunch.* At that point I guess my mind/body had had enough, because the Little Voice (the truth-teller we ignore at our peril) squeaked, *Are you nuts? Can you hear yourself?* From that day on, with only months to retirement, I forced myself to spend the entire lunch period with colleagues, chatting and actually sitting down to eat. I was even able to say, "No I can't help you now, I'm on my way to lunch," to a student who asked for help.

Retirement allowed me one year of getting up early, writing, reading, gardening and enjoying life. Then began the several years of my sister and I trying to do long distance caregiving (three days on, three days off) for our mother so that she could stay in her lovely Victorian apartment in Bordentown, New Jersey, on a beautiful bluff overlooking the Delaware River. A strange bed and being ever alert to my mother's needs, did not make for much sleep; I watched a lot of old movies.

When the time came to wrestle with the awful decision regarding a nursing home, we were pushed in the direction by a friend who had helped care for my mother when we could not be there. "You should see yourselves," she burst out, "I haven't seen a time in the last two years when one or both of you wasn't sick. You are killing yourselves!" And maybe we were, and maybe it had something to do with lack of sleep.

Our bodies were trying to tell us something, but duty and caring spoke louder, as they so often do in women. In my case, symptoms were beginning to appear, but I had no idea what they meant. The two years before my heart's complete collapse were marked by my twice daily visits to my mother in the nursing home ten minutes from my house, as well as eighteen months of trips to doctors who offered sympathy, tests and no diagnosis.

Post-op, my family cracked down on me—one daily visit to my mother, no ifs, ands or buts. So universal was my prohibition that when I showed up one evening, later than my allowed afternoon visit, even the guy who mopped the floors scolded me and sent me home. I did work on getting my rest, but as I have said elsewhere, two cataract surgeries, a colon resection, and my mother's final illness and death did not make that an easy task.

One of my mother's hospice counselors gave me a small set of rules which I still repeat to myself whenever I am tempted to push myself beyond what I know are my limits, whether it is sleep or expending energy. Her name was Alison, and when I have shared them with other women, I am often asked to repeat them so that they can remember them. Alison's Rules are:

Take care of yourself, caregiver or not.

Do what you can (four very powerful words)

No feeling guilty (easier said than done)

What Is Sleep?

Just what constitutes sleep anyway? And how does it connect to heart disease and recovery from heart surgery—or any surgery for that matter. We could start with that quote from Dr. Oz at the top of the chapter. Or we could start with a study quoted by the **Go Red for Women** editors in which researchers found an association between poor sleep and an increase, especially for women, of the inflammation that is a well-known predictor of cardiovascular health.

Interestingly, poor sleep can have a serious effect on our brain health also. An Internet headline by NBC News contributor Barbara Mantel (10/17/2013) proclaims, "A good night's sleep scrubs your brain clean". Researchers at the Center for Translational Neuromedicine at the University of Rochester have discovered that the brain has a unique waste removal system and named it the glymphatic system. It pumps cerebral spinal fluid into the spaces around the brain cells, which are wider when we sleep, and flushes waste into the circulatory system where it makes its way to the liver for processing. It is ten times more active when we sleep, working like a neuronal trash truck, clearing away toxins that have built up when we are awake.

We could also start with my own experience with sleep as I recovered from heart surgery. Initially, all I did was sleep, at least it seemed that way. I would get up, eat, take a nap, do the prescribed exercise, eat, have a nap, read a little, have a nap, eat, watch a funny video and go to bed. No one told me specifically to do this; it just felt like the natural thing to do.

Gradually, as my physical body wanted to be more active, the number of naps decreased, and I went to bed a little later. However, I still got up later, and 10 to 12 hours of sleep was the norm. Actually, given the taxing events during the following year (cataract surgery, colon surgery, care for my mother) I came to believe that for me, this was the norm I would need to follow permanently. Afternoon naps continued, usually for an hour. Gradually, in the second year by now, my need for sleep became a little less as my life became more active and more interesting.

Any upset of the balance, however—too little sleep or too much activity—and I would find myself spending a day or two in bed feeling ill in some nameless way. The lesson was obvious. Sleep was an important factor in maintaining my well-being. Upsetting the balance was sometimes necessary for travel, fun, or life's problems, and had to be planned for or compensated for. It still does.

It is common knowledge that complete deprivation of sleep can lead to the total collapse of both body and mind. What happens when we sleep that makes it such a necessity? Deep in the center of the brain is the pineal gland, which senses when we are exposed to light. The light, even in blind people, enters cells at the back of the eye, forwards it to the occipital lobe in the back of the brain, which sends it on to the pineal gland. This gland is part of the endocrine system, which regulates all kinds of things in our bodies because it produces a substance called melatonin. Think of it this way, says Dr. Oz, "It conducts the symphony of your hormones.[46]

So when the lights go out, and all the discussions of sleep problems advise that the lights must really go out, if you want to get proper sleep. That means no TV, iPhone, or any device that gives off light should be on in your bedroom, which by the way should be used for two things, sleep and sex. If you engage in all kinds of activities in your bed such as working or eating, your brain begins to associate your bed with being awake rather than being asleep. I am fortunate to live in an area with no streetlights, so making a room really dark does not present a problem. For urban dwellers, heavy window coverings are essential for good sleep.

So when we get all the lights out, melatonin levels rise, and tell our bodies to sleep. Our heart rates and blood pressure are lower, our immune systems replenish themselves and at least for the time being, the body's stress response is blocked. We cycle from a light sleep, to moderately deep sleep, to the deepest sleep, which we need to have on a regular basis. The eight or nine hours recommended by most authorities allow for several cycles, and the deep sleep is where we dream, another necessity whether we remember them or not.

All our bodies need this time to refresh and repair, and looking back over my own sleep history, I can see where I did not have healthy sleep habits for many years.

Certainly healthy sleep habits are crucial given the mind and body repair work required after heart surgery. As Dr. Oz says, "Sleep is a serious deal."[47]

A series of studies quoted by Dr. Suzanne Steinbaum have discovered that sleep deprivation decreases the level of leptin, the hormone that tells you when you are full. Thus a lack of proper sleep can lead to over-eating, and undesirable weight gain with no obvious cause. Lack of sleep can also increase blood pressure, and increase the incidence of depression and anger.[48]

Now, because I understand how sleep and rest affect the heart, I try to be responsible.

Gleaned from numerous sources, I try to follow these habits. No TV for an hour or two before bed; having a familiar ritual before bed. In my case, I sit in the kitchen, take my evening pills and chat with my husband. It often becomes a nice time for exchanging thoughts and feelings. The bedroom must be dark. No TV, no work, no electronics—even the green light from the phone must be shut off.

Some ways I have developed to help get me off to dreamland (each of which will be discussed in later chapters) include giving myself a Reiki treatment after I get in bed, imaging a special peaceful place, doing ten rounds of alternate nostril breathing, or just breathing deeply until it feels good. If the Night Owl stays up late, the Night Owl gets up later. If an early day is planned, an early bedtime is a must. Those eight to nine hours are helping to keep me alive.

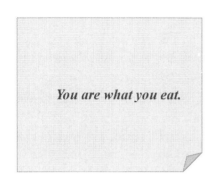

You are what you eat.

11

FOOD

That makes sense. You put food and drink into your mouth; it is absorbed and utilized by various parts of your body, so it really does become "you." As I continue to point out, I am not a medical authority of any kind. I am simply a survivor who has done her homework and can share what she has learned.

Even the authorities don't agree, with public debates about carbs, fat, gluten, etc. Coffee was bad; now it may be helpful. Chocolate seemed inherently evil; now a small portion is recommended. Eggs were bad; now it is okay to eat two a week. There is virtue in red wine, and of course, lots of fruits and vegetables are good, but beware of grapefruit if you take certain medicines.

If even the experts disagree, I can't tell you what to eat. However, I strongly suggest that if you need to reduce or control salt, calories, fat and sugar in your diet, that you begin by consulting your personal physician or a certified nutritionist. The latter can often be found at your local hospital or clinic. What I can tell you is only what I learned about how to regulate my food consumption.

Consider keeping a food diary. If you decide to do this, make it an honest one, no cheating and no skipping. A 6x9 spiral notebook is what I have used. On each right-hand page I mark vertical columns for calories, fat, salt and cholesterol. Above each column I write the amount I am entitled to. Horizontally I divided the page for breakfast, lunch, dinner and bedtime, since I have to take food with my nightly meds.

For example, in the breakfast section I would write all the amounts across the page for cereal, milk and fruit. Lunch? This method began to work for me when I found myself choosing lunches with an eye to being able to write down low numbers. You can also choose a no-fat, low-calorie, low-salt lunch so you can have a little splurge at dinner and not go over your allowed totals. Will you overdo at times? Of course, but no cheating– if you eat it, you write it. When using a food diary it is helpful to average out your weekly totals, so that you can see if you are doing what is best for your heart health.

And where are you supposed to get all this information? There are a variety of charts available both online and in books. I have used the chart in Dean Ornish's first book, *Dean Ornish's Program for Reversing Heart Disease* but it was published in 1996, so you might want to seek out something more recent.

Regardless of what nutritional path you and your health professional choose to follow, keeping a food diary, although a mild nuisance, can get results. I managed to keep a food diary for a year, and it made a difference. I still check labels, but I am familiar enough to structure most meals without looking things up. What about casseroles and stews? That is a bit of work but it can be done, and if you do it right, you'll only have to do it once.

First, separate out each ingredient and tally the numbers for each. Then make a total for the whole dish. It will seem like a humongous amount. Then depending on whether your dish yields six, eight or ten servings, you can divide and get the numbers for one portion. Altering your recipes by using only low salt or salt free broth can help to keep the numbers down. Finally, you can plan what kind of low-number breakfast and lunch you will eat that day to keep your totals down. The next time you make it, just look back in your food diary.

Despite all this diligent record-keeping, we all have our cravings, our split second decisions to give in to them, and the heck with the food charts. Here is where reading labels can help. Not only do they allow you to know exactly what you are putting into your body, they often save me from eating something not good for healthy living. For instance, confronted by the jar of my husband's blue cheese dressing, which I love, and my reasonably tasty cucumber dressing, reading the labels saves me. Comparing 2.5mgs and 14 mgs I am motivated to choose the low fat dressing. Incidentally, these dressing amounts are often given for a two tablespoon portion. I find that one tablespoon is quite enough for me, so I can even cut the 2.5 in half.

When reading labels, two items in your kitchen can be a big help: a set of measuring cups and a set of measuring spoons. When a portion size on the label (and do read the portion size) calls for a half cup, measure it out. After a while you will become accustomed to what that size portion looks like on your plate. Measuring spoons can also help, mostly by showing you how big a tablespoon can be. It is harder to judge the amount, so tablespoons should be used frequently. For example, a measured tablespoon of peanut butter can cover two slices of toast quite adequately, and allow you a small treat without overdoing. And don't forget to write it down.

Most sources agree that pre-packaged foods give the most trouble. Reading labels can help you discern that when the fat is reduced, the sugar and salt are often increased. A "1/3 less salt" label is not much help when there are 900 mgs to start with. Speaking of salt; it is one of my personal cravings. Limits placed on me years ago when I was pregnant have persisted in my not salting pasta water, boiled potatoes, tomatoes and vegetables. One little trick I play on myself usually involves meat. I wait until I have only two or three bites left on my plate and I sprinkle them with a tiny bit of salt—for a treat. In the "No good deed goes unpunished," department, the successful limitation of salt can make you more sensitive to it, especially in restaurants. Once in a while, a dish is too much and a substitution has to be made.

Before my surgery my weight was in normal range. Surviving the surgery cost me twenty pounds. Hooray, I though I'll never have to worry about my weight again. I even had some favorite clothes altered, never thinking that as my life moved toward normal, so would my weight, and beyond normal if I wasn't careful. There have been ups and downs (mostly ups) and I do so miss those brown silk pants that are now too tight to wear. So what I can tell you as a non-authority is choose a dietary plan with your health care professional, write down what you eat, read those labels, and allow yourself a treat once in a while.

The ideas described in this chapter are ones that are part of my life, and my battle is ongoing, just like everyone else. So consult your personal health care provider and/or a certified nutritionist about a plan that is best for you. Then use the diary, the labels and the measuring to make healthful eating a meaningful part of the healing process.

> *"Acupuncture stimulates the release of endorphins, your body's natural pain relievers"*
> Dr. Gary Kaplan, D.O

12

ACUPUNCTURE

When I mentioned to my colon surgeon that acupuncture had eased the abdominal pain from my diverticulitis while I waited for surgery, he looked doubtful. "Do those things, meaning the needles, hurt?" he asked.

I couldn't help smiling. "Of course not. If one hurts you tell the therapist and they take it out." Here we have another example of an experienced, knowledgeable and talented medical professional who knows little about integrative medicine and how it could help his patients. Indeed, a number of needles stuck into one's abdomen, where there is already pain, does not sound like a logical thing to do.

However, these "needles" are as fine as a hair, cause the tiniest zing of sensation when they are inserted, and remain for only about twenty minutes per treatment. They are not the round tubular type we associate with IV's and injections. They are solid, and shaped like a delicate inverted triangle. Inserted along one of the myriad meridian points on the body (see the Energy section) they do not make a hole as such, but push tissue aside to activate the flow of healing energy.

Acupuncture is very old, going back to the ancient Chinese practice of acupressure, done with hands and fingers instead of needles, and still preferred by many even today. The use of needles is a later development. Why and how does this work? Neither research nor medical science has been able to answer that question, except to say that the evidence shows that it does work.

Gary Kaplan, D.O., who directs a chronic pain center in Arlington,

Virginia and is the director of the Medical Acupuncture Research Foundation in Los Angeles, says, "Research shows that acupuncture stimulates the release of endorphins, your body's natural pain relievers, and other research indicates the acupuncture primes your nervous system to keep releasing these pain-blocking endorphins, even when you aren't receiving treatments."

Dr. Kaplan's list of aches and pains relieved by acupuncture treatments in *The Seniors Guide to Pain-Free Living* includes muscle spasms, dental pain, migraines, tension headaches, arthritis, tendinitis, bursitis, wrist ankle and foot problems, irritable bowel syndrome, phantom limb pain and the nausea associated with chemotherapy and anesthesia.[49]

It can be used on an as-needed basis to relieve pain or on a regular basis for a chronic condition. Some use acupuncture as a form of regular practice to maintain general health by balancing energy flow. Pain relief is usually emphasized in Western practice and research. As a general way to maintain health, it is most often used in Eastern medical practice.

I began to see a Chinese acupuncturist who was also an M.D., during the eighteen months before my cardiac train wreck when no one could seem to figure out what was wrong with me. It did help me to feel a bit better in a general way. During the first two treatments, I could feel the movement of rearranged energy flowing in my body.

When, in the Fall of 2007, colon surgery loomed, I decided with the surgeon's permission, to delay it until January of 2008. Once again I turned to acupuncture, and thus the needles in the abdomen. Later, during the "Battle of the Statins," I used it for the joint pain, and it did not provide relief, so I discontinued it.

As Dr. Kaplan and others have said, it does not always work for a person or a condition. He recommends that if after ten treatments no relief is evident, treatment should be stopped.[50]

So what should one expect when trying this healing modality? Asking the usual questions about training, years of practice and licensing in your state, is always wise when dealing with a medical professional. An MD or a licensed acupuncturist will always take a good medical history. My Chinese M.D. also examined my tongue at each visit and checked my pulse, or pulses as per Chinese medicine.

One lies on a padded table, or sometimes sits in a special chair for work on the back. Usually only the necessary clothing is removed or pushed aside. Needles may be inserted in what seems like odd places—such as in the calf for blood pressure—but this is all done according to the charts of energy meridians which are centuries old.

I would then be left alone with soothing music for about twenty minutes. Sometimes I came close to falling asleep. On return, the needles were removed and discarded. If you encounter a practitioner who re-uses needles, even if they claim to sterilize them—do not return to that office.

Currently I am not seeing an acupuncturist regularly, but should the need arise, I would not hesitate to make use of this healing practice. The answer to my ever-skeptical, "Does this stuff work?" is once again in the affirmative.

> *"You don't have to be able to put your foot behind your head or move away to an ashram. If you can breathe, you can practice yoga."*
> Tara Stiles in
> *Yoga Cures/Intent Blog*

13

YOGA

"Oh I could never twist myself into all those pretzel shapes!" is a common response when I suggest that someone, especially a heart surgery survivor, give yoga a try. Not a surprising response when most photos one sees are of extreme poses which, let's face it, often resemble pretzels. And in many ads for yoga classes, one reads the strange sounding names— Ashtanga, Bikram, Kundalini, Inyegar, Vinyasa, Hatha.

In Sanskrit, the word means "union," and the union/balance of mind/body/spirit is the goal of Yoga practice. Yoga has been around, as far as we know, for about 5,000 years, and it does come in an almost endless variety of schools. The names can add to the image of a strange and exotic activity, not for the ordinary person. Not so.

My experience with yoga serves as a template for all the healing modalities I have made use of in the past years. I began, as I always do, with "Does this stuff work?" The difference is that in yoga, satisfying my curiosity took place many years ago. I began with a teacher of Hatha yoga— for health and energy, not intended as a necessarily spiritual practice. This enabled many community members to enjoy the physical benefits of yoga while not having to commit to a spiritual practice. I likened it to learning to dance, or to skate. You follow the steps very mechanically until you master them; then you can feel them go "click" and do them without thinking about it. The teacher was gentle but very meticulous, and each posture was worked to completion with a great deal of individual help

Next, I worked with the members of the Kripalu Ashram, which was located nearby (they have since moved to Connecticut) and learned that there are different ways to do the same postures. I also had several classes with teachers who were not really concerned with doing postures correctly. I had already learned that if not done properly, the postures, or asanas, do not give much benefit. I soon left those classes.

During the eighteen months when my heart problems were misdiagnosed, when no one seemed to know what was wrong with me, I worked with a therapeutic yoga class. Here we used blankets and blocks to create release for some fairly extreme postures; but they did make me feel better. Once the initial recovery period from my heart surgery was over, I asked both my primary and my cardiologist if it was safe to go back to yoga, and if there were any postures I should avoid, like shoulder stands.

And here is illustrated the problem this book hopes to address. These well-meaning physicians could not help me, because they knew little or nothing about yoga. In attempting to be a responsible patient, which I always do, I was left on my own to make decisions about an aspect on integrative medicine which I had found very helpful for many years, pre-surgery. Fortunately for me, the Cardiac Rehab program at my local Wellness Center, which is supervised by the hospital, offers both chair yoga and gentle floor yoga, both approved for heart patients.

Yes, in most classes you will sit on the floor on a rectangular mat, sometimes assisted by blocks or blankets. But there is such a thing as chair yoga, which is ideal for those whose age or health issues make getting up and down from the floor too difficult. You can find information about chair yoga by Googling it. As someone who practiced floor yoga for many years, I can attest to the amazing number of modified poses one can do in a chair. I have been in such a class, with people who have back, knee, arthritis and age issues. The oldest member was 93, and one of our instructors was 90! According to the Guinness Book of Records, the world's oldest documented yoga teacher is 91-year-old Bernice Bates of Pinellas Park, Florida, who says, "I think yoga is the best exercise there is. It is for everybody." (Lisa Flam TODAY.com contributor)

There are gentle floor and chair classes at many Y's and health centers, since yoga has not only become popular, but highly recommended for heart patients. Virtually every source in my list of helpful books cited the following benefits: Regular practice of yoga can:

- reduce arthritis pain
- reduce stress hormones—very important
- increase flexibility—crucial in improving balance and preventing falls
- lower blood pressure and heart rate—need we say more?
- increase relaxation hormones—serotonin, dopamine and endorphins

But not everyone has access to this type of program. Caution is necessary when choosing a class and a teacher. For any class you choose to explore, be sure that the instructor is certified. Ask if you can visit a class to see if it is right for you. "Listen to and honor your body," and "Do only what you can," are phrases you should hear. If it seems that the instructor is pushing people into extreme or painful poses, move on.

However, most beginning classes, especially Hatha yoga, are usually quite simple and allow you to take it only as far as you want to go. Are the results worth it? For me, they certainly are. After a yoga class, I feel both relaxed and energized. Physical and mental kinks have been ironed out. In concentrating on breathing, or creating a posture/pose/asana, your mind gets too busy to worry about your life, and that is why you relax.

Breathing properly is a major part of yoga. If you do not seem to be expert right away, give your body time to adjust. It may take a little while if you are not accustomed to really filling your lungs entirely with oxygen. You will learn to appreciate the benefits of the so-called belly breathing for both relaxation and increased energy. That is because yoga does not only help you to relax and stretch, to heal and soothe your aches and pains away. Filling your whole body's cells with the oxygen supplied by deep breathing also increases your post-yoga energy.

My class is on Monday, and besides the relaxation/guided imagery with which we end the class, I usually am able to fit in a nap. When I was working full-time I had an evening class, and it was a lovely prelude to a restful night's sleep.

In my world, Tuesday is an interesting day. My energy level is noticeably higher—a good thing. However, I have a tendency to over-exert myself as a result—not so good. It is not an exaggeration to say that I have to be careful not to undertake too many tasks on the day after my class. It is all part of the discipline I have had to adopt as part of my healing.

So even if it seems that you are too stiff and out of shape, give chair or gentle floor yoga a chance. The breathing and slow stretching may loosen you up more than you ever expected. Tara Stiles, in her yoga blog *Yoga Cures*, says it well. "You are your own best teacher, healer, and inspiration. It all starts with a deep breath. Yoga can cure most of life's aches and pains from back pain, anxiety, sleeping problems migraines and more; and what it doesn't end up curing, it helps us deal with a whole lot better."

Many times I have lamented, "I wish I could find a cardiologist who does yoga!" Imagine my delight when I interviewed my own heart surgeon for this book about healing modalities. Dr. James McClurkin related that heart surgeons often develop back problems from standing in odd positions for long periods of time, and that when it happened to him, he used yoga to find relief. He also encouraged me to try more vigorous forms if I wished, that was perfectly okay.

For those of the, "I don't have time," persuasion, what you learn in a yoga class can easily be incorporated in small bits into your daily life. Before getting into bed, a session of ten deep yoga breaths can help you to relax into sleep. So can alternate nostril breathing, easy to learn in any basic yoga class. Combined with some imagery and/or Reiki (more about those later) you have a wonderful prescription for dreamland after a busy day.

In the morning, I have found that doing some yoga moves before getting up is both a time saver and a help in undoing morning stiffness. While the body is warm anyway, things are easier. Hand exercises work well for arthritis. Toes, ankles and knees can be awakened that much more easily. Lying on my side I can stretch out my hip joints and my back.

I am fortunate to have a lovely view of grass and trees out my bathroom window, and I try to remember to pause, admire the beauty, chant an OHM or two to start the day. As the day goes on, just sitting quietly and taking a few deep breaths can give a nice lift to your energy and your spirits.

On pages 112 and 113 of the *Readers Digest Family Guide to Natural Medicine* there is a series of stretches, many of which are variations on yoga postures, which can be done at your desk, if that is where you must spend your day.

It may not be a yoga posture, but a new book recommends simply standing up every twenty minutes. The author does phone calls and opens mail in this position—another way to fit healing motions into a busy life.

Of course, going on to more advanced yoga classes and postures is always an option. You too, may one day achieve "pretzel" status. But for anyone of any age or physical condition, some form of basic yoga is a boon for lessening stress and fostering a healthy and flexible body for a long life.

"The arrival of a good clown exercises more beneficial influence upon the health of a town than twenty asses laden with drugs."
Thomas Sydenham, a 17th Century Physician

14

LAUGHTER/ HUMOR/CARING

Remember that my family understood from the earliest days of my recovery that I needed to laugh. After coming home on December 18, I received for Christmas the entire set of "Are You Being Served," the British sitcom that we had all watched over and over because it made us laugh, even when we had all but memorized the dialogue. Each evening after supper I was escorted to the computer for a half hour of amusement, until I had watched the entire series.

Our extended family has always had a wacky sense of humor. My late father was a master teller of jokes and stories, complete with appropriate accents. On the night of his burial, our tiny apartment rocked with laughter as my uncles retold the favorites they had learned from him. Several recounted that retelling his stories helped them through the terrors of WWII. It was a warm September evening and the windows were open. I wondered what the neighbors might think about all the laughing. Then I realized what my father might think. He would have asked no finer legacy than healing laughter.

As I dug into various books in my search for healing, it was no surprise to find "laughter" and "humor" in almost all the indexes. In *YOU: Staying Young,* Dr. Oz advises learning how to tell a good joke as part of your healing. "There's lots of evidence that a good laugh can help improve your immune system, and humor can also have a valuable effect on your memory."[51]

In addition he says, "When we laugh, natural killer cells that destroy tumors and viruses increase…Laughing lowers blood pressure, increases oxygen in the body with deeper respirations, and helps to address the effect of mental stress on the arteries. And you can't beat the price."[52]

Editor Bill Gottlieb of *Prevention Magazine* recommends, "Make time for a daily chuckle. A good laugh triggers the release of endorphins, chemicals in the brain that produce feelings of euphoria. It also suppresses the production of cortisol."[53] You remember cortisol.

"Exercise your funny bone," advises Robert N. Jamison, PhD, of the pain management program at Brigham and Women's Hospital in Boston. "Laughter is a powerful weapon against pain. Laughter can renew your sense that life is worth living."[54] He suggests posting cartoons on the fridge, collecting funny videos to play on bad days. I would add keep a supply of CDs which make you feel upbeat. The Beach Boys and Charleston music do it for me.

In *From the Heart,* Kathy Kastan, psychologist and heart surgery survivor says, "Read the comics. Cultivate relationships with people who make you laugh. Believe it or not, laughter is good for your heart."[55]

Health guru Andrew Weil, *in Healthy Aging,* cites his mother's ability to see the ridiculous side of things as the key to her long life. "The absurdities that can make you laugh in the midst of misfortune…especially in the midst of misfortune."[56] He also relates the story of Dr. Madan Kataria of Mumbai, India, who travels the world teaching a practice called laughing yoga. He gets groups of people together to laugh for fifteen or twenty minutes as a physical and mental exercise.

"You should be laughing till it hurts, as opposed to giggling. Want a home remedy? Forget the bowl of chicken soup and watch the Marx Brothers *Duck Soup*, says Robin Dunbar, PhD and Oxford psychologist in the *AARP Magazine*.[57]

Taking a cue from little kids can't hurt either, according to Dr. Stephen Sinatra, "Children laugh on an average of four hundred times a day; adults only fifteen."[58] He quotes a study from the University of California at Loma Linda in which two groups of heart attack survivors had equal rehab. One group watched a funny video every day. After a year, the comedy watchers had lower stress hormones, lower blood pressure, needed fewer meds, and had healthier electrocardiograms. They had two heart attacks compared to the ten in the control group.

And, of course, there is Norman Cousins, who laughed his way to a cure for a mysterious disease for which conventional doctors could offer no hope. As a result of his best-selling book, *The Anatomy of an Illness*, there are now laughter therapies in and out of the more progressive hospitals. Thanks to a film starring Robin Williams, many people are now aware of the Gesundheit Institute, where the real Patch Adams is devoted to using humor to alleviate a variety of ailments.

My own surgeon is a great fan of laughter. "I was the class clown in high school, but in med school they asked me to tone it down. Nobody wants a smart-aleck surgeon. But the glass-half-full people laugh more, and live longer." He is glad to see, "A family kid around with a patient; it's a lot more fun for everybody"

His partner, Dr. Guerati, a European gentleman, had a humorous comment each time he visited me. On the day of my discharge he announced, with mock seriousness, "There is a gentleman downstairs asking for you. It seems he wants to take you home with him. Do you know anything about that?" I was happy to reply, "If he's handsome, send him up."

Which brings me to my encounter with a hospital clown. You will recall the poem, "Chuckles and the Afternoon TEE." That he offered amusement and comfort to both adults and children made me want to meet him. I tracked him down through the hospital and we met over coffee in a fast food restaurant. Dave Stoudt turned out to be very ordinary man in his sixties, who has been Chuckles for thirty-five years. After retiring from marketing positions with a local oil company, he drove a school bus for a while. Currently he is a bus driver for an assisted living facility, taking elderly residents on trips to cheer their days.

Beginning when he saw how many people came to cheer his young son when he had to spend Christmas in the hospital, Dave cast about for something he could do. "There were enough Santas," he explains, "So I hit on being a clown." A member of his church made the first costume, and a friend offered to help, so there were two Chuckles.

The visits have grown from one children's ward to eight hospitals, adults, and over a thousand bears. That hospitalized boy has joined them, and now there are three Chuckles.

Family members gather each year—they have expanded to three

109

generations—to pack and deliver the bears. Several stuffed animal companies provide bears at a deep discount, and money is raised via a mailing list of generous donors.

Stories abound, of the "Biggest smile you could imagine," from a cancer patient; families in neonatal units who are comforted by his visit; special needs children in an Easter Seals facility; even psychiatric hospitals. "Everybody loves a teddy bear." The good feelings (which have to be good for hearts all around) keep spreading out. Dave's church now has a Bear Tree, where members attach donated bears. And when the visits are over, the whole team has a big party at one member's barn.

Of his job driving the bus for assisted living, Chuckles says, "I love to help people. These folks are going down the home stretch and I want to make it as special as I can." All that good feeling has to be good for hearts.

In the spirit of not taking things too seriously, but getting a life-saving job done, readers should check out the following website www.DayofDance.com. This is a website which features a catchy modern tune, the lyrics of which are the symptoms of a woman's heart attack. Hospital staffs all over the country were enlisted to sing and dance this song. Doctors, nurses, technicians, secretaries were all happy to make fools of themselves in order to teach women these danger signs. It is wonderful serious fun.

And from my own experience, I offer the following poem:

SHE JESTS AT SCARS

The forty-year hysterectomy
scar lies smooth and flat
a tiny line from navel on down.

The broken-open sternum
is wired back together.
They have promised me
I won't go off in airports.

The long tidy chest scar
admits me to the exclusive
Zipper Club. We pull
our blouses down like
lodge brothers shaking hands
to validate our membership,
which includes extra cleavage.

In between, I'm sporting three
portholes from the chest drains,
triple ovals–like a 50's Buick
Roadmaster–they were
top-of-the-line back then.

Am I status-y and glamorous at last?

Another View Of Scars

Humor aside, it needs to be acknowledged that for some women, scarring isn't funny.

When you see the jacket photograph of Kathy Kastan on her book *From the Heart: A Woman's Guide to Living Well with Heart Disease,* you know she doesn't think that the subject of scars is funny. The president of *WomanHeart:* The National Coalition for Women with Heart Disease, as she poses with her white blouse open to the waist, revealing her own surgical scar, it is obvious that she takes the subject seriously. She comments:

Some women heart patients have scars from surgery that effect how they see themselves. Let's face it, they are not pretty. But you have nothing to be embarrassed or ashamed about. If that's how you feel, try to turn your thinking around. Give yourself time for your scars to heal. Eventually, they'll become a part of you just like your freckles or wrinkles. Try to think of each scar as a badge of courage—like battle scars—or as a symbol of your ability to survive.[59]

I haven't known how to explain my attitude toward scars until recently. The ones described in the poem are quite real, but their appearance just doesn't bother me. A low-cut top is fine. It shows my scar–so what? And bikinis never were my style. Do I consider them a badge of honor? Maybe. On a Canadian website run by heart attack survivor Carolyn Thomas, called Heart Sisters, there is a wonderful quote: "Never be ashamed of your scar. It simply means that you are stronger than whatever tried to hurt you."[http://myheartsisters.org/2012/10/26/love-your-scars].

This website quotes women's views about their scars ranging from actually believing that "I can't wear this shirt because it shows," (as if there might be a law against it!) and "I'm not at the point where I can look at it as a battle scar. I wear high-neck tops even in the summer," to "They are my battle scars earned and gloriously celebrated as such," and "A scar is never ugly. We must see all scars as beauty. Because take it from me, a scar does not form on the dying. A scar means I survived!"

Thomas' website, which has been called the best heart blog on the web, is the result of her own heart disease, and training at the Mayo Clinic. With her unique perspective she offers information for the general public, heart patients and family members, and health professionals. The site is independent and self-funded. Many of the items are completely frank opinions from female heart patients all around the world. An example of this frankness is a page titled, "Stupid Things Doctors Say to Women Heart Patients." It has thirty-three global entries. If you have been misdiagnosed, you will enjoy it.

I am blessed with a husband who teases me that I am a "good-looking old broad," dressed or undressed. So much for my self-centered view. My research has showed me a very different picture, and helped to explain why I have the luxury of jesting at my scars. I am now aware that not all partners take scarring in stride. I do know of one husband who does. When his wife finally got up the courage to tell him how she worried that her scars from multiple cancer surgeries would come between them, he replied, "When I look at those scars they simply remind me how lucky we both are that you survived."

I have been, unknown to me, spared two things which might have prevented any joking around. The first is pain. There was very little pain in the early weeks, aside from a muscle spasm in my back. It may be partly because I was absolutely meticulous about following the instructions with which I was sent home. Our hospital even provided detailed directions for getting a t-shirt off without actually raising the arms overhead–a no-no for a wired together chest.

The only significant pain (aka pain that requires a call to the doctor) appeared several months after the surgery. As all us survivors know, it can be hard to distinguish between a possible heart attack and left chest pain. In my case, after the required visit to the doctor, it turned out to be from nerves re-growing and making repairs, and a change in the way the heart was positioned in my chest. As long as I knew what it was, I could deal with it until it worked itself out.

It took me a number of the early weeks to roll over on my left side, literally inching my way one night at a time; not from pain but just the fear of damaging something. When I finally achieved my goal, I discovered that it was a place where, with the proper adjustment of the pillow, I could actually relax and fall asleep. Even now, I sometimes have mild discomfort in this position, which is relieved by rolling over on my back and taking a few deep breaths.

There was a second problem from which I was spared also. With the sternum wired together, there are sometimes very real problems that can develop and should be reported to your doctor immediately. The same is true of the scar. If it is particularly lumpy or otherwise unpleasant in appearance, and this really bothers you, there are procedures which can sometimes improve it. The bottom line is that if there are any problems, do not suffer in silence. You are not being vain or silly. Talk to your doctor promptly. If the scar is a serious issue between you and a partner, perhaps some counseling would help to resolve things for both of you.

Speaking of vain and silly, I will confess to what really does strike me as definitely unfunny. As an aging woman, the crepe-like skin on my arms does not make me write humorous poems. It makes me lament to myself, "Whose arms are these? They can't possibly be mine!" But they are, and there is nothing I can do about them but be grateful every day that I am still here to complain about them.

> *"Exercise, exercise, exercise. It's the only wonder drug we have."*
> Dr. Roseanne Leipzig,
> Mt. Sinai School of Medicine

15

EXERCISE

Of all the healing modalities which are known to improve overall health as well as aid in recovery, exercise in some form tops all the lists. It is also the one that is most difficult to get people to do, especially women. Why is this so? It could be because it is not associated with pleasant feelings.

Yoga relaxes, as do reflexology, massage, healing music, Reiki, meditation, even laughter. But exercise means effort, the physical use of the body, and too many people believe that joining a gym means wearing spandex tights on a not-so-good-looking figure among skinny twenty-somethings. No wonder only one fifth of cardiac patients even try cardiac rehabilitation programs.

I never thought I'd become a gym rat—all that spandex, all those grim body builders, buff, tough, determined. Zombie-faced watchers of the ever-present TV, I believed, they pedal, pedal, pump, pump, lift, lift, impossible weights for impossible times. That was before seven hours of heart surgery.

That was also before, as per the instructions from my doctors, I spent 12 weeks in the Cardiac Rehab program at my local hospital and entered a long-term program (read the rest of my life) at a local Wellness Center, sponsored by the hospital. I am now a dedicated gym rat, but my stereotypical image of gyms is long gone.

I am now quite familiar with treadmills, elliptical trainers, rowing machines and a host of other devices I would have once turned my back on as too boring to bother. But as a weak-kneed patient recovering from massive heart surgery, I welcomed any activity which would help me to get well again. That is how I discovered two essential things: support from a knowledgeable staff and the camaraderie of other survivors are essential factors in recovery. A while later, an online headline from Cardio Smart, the web site of the American College of Cardiology (7/9/2009) caught my eye:

CARDIAC REHABILITATION SAVES LIVES

It detailed how several major universities have conducted studies to demonstrate that after a cardiac event, cardiac rehab can substantially increase survival rates (Duke University) with supervised aerobic exercise (Brandeis University and The University of Vermont) yoga (Emory University School of Medicine) and talk therapy (Washington University at St. Louis). This is true regardless of clinical diagnosis, gender, race, socioeconomic background, even advanced age.

At Brandeis, several hundred thousand patients were followed for five years and cardiac rehab improved survival rates from 21 to 34 percent. Indeed the small percentage of the very elderly who participated in the study obtained especially large gains. The Duke study was one of the first big efforts to show that people who attend all 36 sessions of rehab (which is what Medicare pays for) were less likely to die in the next three or four years.

It isn't just the cardiologists. A quick perusal of the Internet can yield headlines like the following.

EXERCISE MAY HELP PREVENT DEPRESSION LATER IN LIFE—
University of Toronto study.

ACTIVITY LINKED TO LESS AGE-RELATED BRAIN CHANGE—
study published in journal *Neurology.*

TOO MUCH SITTING LINKED TO CARDIOVASCULAR DISEASE—
Runner's World.

*FITNESS IN MIDDLE AGE REDUCES HEART FAILURE RISK—***Go Red For Women.**

Information like this would cause any survivor of a cardiac event to head for the nearest rehab facility, right? Not necessarily. According to the American Heart Association, only a small portion of survivors exercise, despite their doctor's urging; many don't follow through, and far too many of them are women.

Local hospitals all over the country offer, and Medicare pays for, programs of carefully monitored exercises for twelve weeks. After that, there are a variety of programs at local YMCA's and health clubs.

So what is the problem? According to one news article, cardiac rehab conjures up images of "old people dragging around on treadmills." As a member of the Wellness Center's CR gang, I can assert that we may be seniors, but we are not dragging, and we do not spend all our time on treadmills. We validate what the university studies are showing.

We have decided that life is worth living and we are willing to do what it takes to live it well. We are open heart surgery survivors like me; others have pacemakers, heart attacks, stents. We trade jokes, rehash last night's game and tease our therapists. We agree that no matter how awful we feel when we get up; if we come here, the supportive atmosphere helps us to feel better physically, mentally and emotionally. One of us showed up recently in a Hogwarts t-shirt, so I guess we even believe in magic.

The clinical name for what we do for each other is "psycho-social support". Informally, it's the "been-there-done-that" effect. Just as exercise is universally valued, so is emotional support, no matter what we call it. In the *Seniors Guide to Pain-Free Living* Dr. David Spiegel, Director of the Complementary Medicine Clinic at Stanford University's School of Medicine says, "Psycho-social support is so valuable that it should be an essential component of medical treatment…it allows people to stop putting up a front, which drains energy, and share feelings. Sometimes regular friends shy away from illness, and may fade out of the picture."[60]

Drs. Efteriades and Coulin-Glaser in *The Woman's Heart-an Owner's Manual,* are more specific, "Depression is common especially in women, after heart surgery,"[61] and "Cardiac rehab is important after a heart attack, placement of a stent, valve surgery or coronary bypass surgery."[62] They add that such programs should include exercise, patient education, lifestyle modifications, and psychological support to accomplish these goals.

According to cardiologist Mimi Guarneri in T*he Heart Speaks,* "Research has documented the healing powers of group support by Dean Ornish, among others. Helping to express feelings, members also find encouragement for lifestyle changes like exercise, diet and smoking cessation."[63]

We can lift each other's spirits when the pace of recovery seems all too slow. Standing around waiting to use the blood pressure machine, three of us overheard a new member lamenting the pressure he felt from his too-devoted wife, who was monitoring every morsel he ate on his now limited diet. "I'm tempted to just give up and eat anything I want again!" We whirled around as a group, "No! You must not give up." A few minutes of group "counseling" and we had encouraged him. We also got our therapist to agree to have a talk with his wife.

There is a retired math professor with whom I exchange news of cultural events and bad puns. A former aeronautical engineer in his eighties, who lives in a farmhouse he heats with wood he chops himself, challenges us with questions from "Are You Smarter Than a Fifth Grader?" Need to discuss military history with those who were there? Take your choice of WWII, Korea, Vietnam, or Desert Storm. Keeping up with the pop scene? The father of a major rock star has exercised with us. We even have a retired cardiologist among our companions. True, one man walks a bit slowly on his treadmill, but he had a heart transplant at Penn six years ago.

The women's numbers are, as the university studies also show, much smaller than the men. Currently they include a psychologist, a retired food service worker, a massage therapist, a teacher, a writer, a retired nurse, a singer, a physicist, and a young mother with two sons. Our oldest, at ninety-one, was a sergeant in the Women's Army Corps (WAC) in WWII.

Why don't more women follow up on what is obviously a way to restore a healthy functioning lifestyle? A surprising number of them take care of grandchildren. Older women, who heart patients tend to be, may just think exercise is for younger people. But one widow in her eighties, with a very trim figure, has said. "Since coming here I lost two dress sizes, a bra size and a shoe size." In my own case, regular exercise specifically suited to my needs, has helped to restore my heart function to near normal, in spite of medical setbacks which caused me to restart my program entirely, several times.

It is even possible to find romance. The lady whose clothing sizes changed paired with a widowed fellow exerciser when they found that they had much in common. In their middle eighties, they "keep company" for weekly movies, family outings, and even occasionally go dancing.

We are offered a class in chair yoga, specially formulated for recovering patients. After years of floor yoga, I am amazed at how many postures can be done in a chair. Our class has an international flavor with people of Hispanic, Pilipino and Asian backgrounds—not to mention the man who sports a different humorous t-shirt at each class. Our teacher, who has long years of experience, is 65 and has two replaced hips. Her substitute is 90 and puts us through a challenging workout when she appears.

Presiding over all this is our exercise physiologist, encourager-in-chief, positive enforcer, Dave Woods, guaranteed to make you smile. His able assistants Lindsey, Suzanne, Kendra, Tyler and Megan do the same. New folks arrive, some weak and not too cheerful. Within weeks they are moving forward, no matter how slowly, at a pace suited to their needs; and they are smiling.

But does it have to be a supervised program? Others describe gardening, hiking, biking and even dancing as keeping up their spirits and their physical condition. Dr. Stanley Hazen, preventive and cardiology and rehabilitation chief at the Cleveland Clinic commented that, "It can be just a brisk walk, or swimming, or a stationary bike. That's the key: find something you like and are willing to do."

In my case, walking and gardening are my additional activities. With a tool loaned by the Wellness Center, I measured off my small dead-end street and the cul-de-sac opposite. Two trips up and back and I have walked a mile after supper, said hello to the neighbors, and admired the sunset. In winter, daytime walking, well bundled up, is best.

As for gardening, day-long sessions with bushes, trees and flowers, was my habit pre-surgery. Now, roughly an hour is what I do, usually one job planned in advance. Then I sit on my patio and admire my work, trying not to fuss about what must be left for another day.

According to my heart surgeon, Dr. James McClurkin, of the Doylestown Hospital Heart Institute, we are increasingly realizing that mental activity is equally important for a healthy recovery. Many authors mention the same two ways to keep depression at bay and cheer yourself up—get a computer and learn a new language. The computer can connect you socially (as well as allow you to write a book) after you survive the ordeal of learning to use it. Hint: seek out a 12-year-old to help you if you do not have a tech-savvy spouse. Learning a new language can provide tremendous stimulation to the "little grey cells."

Mental activity for me includes active participation in the poetry community of Bucks County with classes and readings, free-lance writing for a weekly newspaper, writing fiction, the ubiquitous daily crossword, and being a news junkie of long standing.

However, others find mental or social stimulation in crafts. One retired nursing director took up painting and is winning awards. Another takes regular courses at the local community college. Making music alone or in groups can be very satisfying. Volunteering in a variety of ways, from the local hospital to ushering at a local theater can get you out of the house on a regular basis. There is also doing family history research—the list goes on, and it keeps you going. One woman, a confessed "phone gabber" keeps her stationary bike next to the phone, and all that time chatting is also spent exercising.

In her *Heart Book*, Dr. Suzanne Steinbaum presents a sometimes whimsical list of suggestions for exercise. If you golf, walk and carry your clubs. Take the stairs whenever you can. Wear sneakers and walk anywhere you can: the mall, the park or walk to work. Do squats in the kitchen while cooking. Do leg lifts while knitting. Put on some music and dance. Dr. Steinbaum did it, feeling cooped up at home with a small baby—she danced with the baby. She concludes with the classic, "Move it or lose it."[64]

As always, if you are going out on a program of your own, get your cardiologist's permission, and keep in touch with your regular checkups. In terms of research, I can say that every source I consulted about recovery from, or even avoidance of, heart disease strongly recommends exercise.

To quote Dr. McClurkin, "We can't cure people of heart disease, but we can change their survival curve." He is adamant that, "The single biggest factor in how well you do after surgery is staying active. Both your mind and body have to be doing something."

If you or a loved one is a cardiac patient, especially a woman, put aside your image of what cardiac rehab is. Consider joining a supervised exercise program because that headline was accurate: Cardiac Rehab Saves Lives. Let one of them be yours

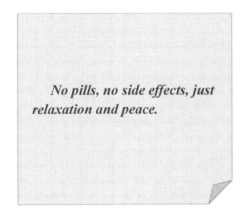

No pills, no side effects, just relaxation and peace.

16

MASSAGE

I became a devotee of massage therapy long before my heart surgery. An injury to my right trapezius muscle (caused by my own stupidity in not moving properly out of a shoulder stand in a yoga class) left me with pain and problems all down my right arm. A program at a gym made it worse. With my usual skeptical approach to alternative therapies, I was hesitant to try massage. But with five months of pain, and trust in the judgment of a friend who is a physical therapist in her own right, I agreed to make an appointment with Marge.

Since then, people have said to me, "Oh, I couldn't let anyone touch me in that way." I guess I felt a little of that at my first session. After all, taking all your clothes off is always a bit of an adventure. But I was lying face up, modestly covered by a sheet, on a very comfortable table, with a gentle smiling woman about my own age asking me to describe my problem. It wasn't all that nervous-making.

An hour later, after I had turned over and she had worked mostly on my back, I was hooked. She used a technique called trigger point, where pressure is patiently applied to the knotted muscle, causing it to let go. The knot which had plagued me for months had finally let go. However Marge warned, it would most likely come back a few more times. It did, and I developed a routine of monthly massages over several years, for relaxation. We chatted while she worked, about many things besides healing.

An excellent source for information, with color illustrations about all aspects of holistic/integrative medicine is *The Reader's Digest Family*

Guide to Natural Medicine—How to Stay Healthy the Natural Way. Yes, I was surprised too, having thought of *Reader's Digest* as a publication with fairly conservative views. Under massage, the index lists 39 items for using massage for various problems. If you want to actually see what a massage looks like, there are color photographs starting on page 157. This informative book covers healing therapies from all over the world.

When Marge decided to return to graduate school, she did what I suppose is rather unusual for any therapist. She booked a massage for herself with all the local practitioners whom she respected, and sent each of her clients to the one she felt was most suited to their needs. I drew Mary Ellen.

An amazing woman, she is a talented practitioner of massage, reflexology (a form of foot massage) and Reiki. Though legally blind from macular degeneration, she has managed a college degree, a house, a husband, two sons, two dogs and a cat, as well as being an ordained Inter-Faith minister and a member of a local a capella singing group. She has also survived a double mastectomy for breast cancer.

Who she is as a person is as inspiring as her therapeutic talents. She explains it this way: "I am not a blind person. I am Mary Ellen, who happens to be blind. Outside of driving a car, there is very little I cannot do if I want to take the trouble to master it." Keeping up with the world via a voice computer; she confounds me with all the latest books she has read on tape. It is she who helped to point me in the direction of excellent sources for healing modalities.

So, what about massage? In the *Senior's Guide to Pain-Free Living,* it has been defined as, "the systematic and purposeful manipulation of the soft tissues of the body." The manipulation can vary from gentle to vigorous—kneading, pressing, rubbing, stroking, rolling and tapping.[65] Coming under the general heading of body work, it can take many forms; some take place fully clothed, some not. They range from the forceful manipulations of Rolfing; through Alexander Technique which concentrates on the spine; to Shiatsu, which seeks to balance energy forces in the body; to Rubenfeld Synergy which combines talk therapy with gentle touch; to the deep touch of Swedish massage; to more gentle forms for various chronic conditions.

There is also a form called seated massage, done fully clothed in a special chair. It is useful for back and neck problems, and can easily be fitted in on a lunch hour. My experience has been at the lower end of the scale, with Swedish massage, but I have a friend who swears by Rolfing. Self-massage is another helpful technique. Often known as Do In, it is actually possible to give yourself a refreshing head-to-toe massage with your own hands. I was introduced to this form by my current chair yoga teacher, but directions can be found in *New Choices in Natural Healing*. Illustrated directions begin on page 572. This source is filled with directions for many healing therapies; I recommend it highly if you are curious, but do not have experience yet.

Trust in the therapist is essential. How does one find a competent and trustworthy person? Word of mouth is probably the best method; ask around and you may be surprised at how many people enjoy massage. Hearing the experience of someone you trust can be helpful. Some of the more enlightened hospitals can be a source of referrals. Thankfully, the image of the sleazy "massage parlor" is slowly fading away, as well qualified professionals advertise in dignified ways. Ads in local health publications can sometimes provide leads, but initially, caution is advised, to make sure of several things. This is advisable with any health practitioner, even an MD.

First, the person should be well qualified. Ask about certifications. There is the American Massage Therapy Association, and there may be state and local licensing requirements. Ask about years of experience, and the exact type of massage offered. Do not be shy about asking about fees; but remember, if this person is a qualified professional, he or she is entitled to earn a living with this skill. I currently pay $75.00 for a one hour session.

The person's personality should also suit you. Is gender an issue? It is for me; I prefer a female masseuse, but both of my therapists have male clients. I did not have the following problem, but I know others who have experienced it. If there is anything about the therapist's "touch" which does not suit you, move on to another choice. You may also want to try different kinds of massage until you find one which suits your needs.

Benefits? According to Janet Kahn, PhD, senior research scientist at Wellsley College Center for Research on Women in Tacoma Park, Maryland, in *The Senior's Guide to Pain-Free Living,* studies at major hospitals and universities have shown that the various forms of massage can relive symptoms of fibromyalgia, chronic fatigue syndrome, back pain, cancer and high blood pressure. The various forms of body work, especially the gentler forms, can lower blood pressure, (a boon for a heart patient like me), strengthen the immune system, lower cortisol levels, improve symptoms of anxiety and depression. Kahn cites further studies that show a reduction in stress hormones in HIV patients. Massage also hastens the elimination of toxic wastes such as uric acid and lactic acid that are stored in the muscles.[66]

As an example of combining therapies, Mary Ellen uses music as an adjunct to a treatment. Marge and I usually chatted while she worked and that was also enjoyable; we found we had a lot in common. As soon as I could rest comfortably on my stomach after the surgery, I returned to regular massage, and continue to this day. It is just one more element to use in the journey toward your own healing, whatever your problem happens to be.

> *"I believe that sound,*
> *especially music, can be a great*
> *healer."*
> Steven Halpern, PhD

17

MUSIC AND OTHER SOUNDS

We have all heard that old saw, "Music hath charms to soothe the savage breast." Since ancient times various kinds of chants and songs have been used by healers to relieve suffering. Nowhere is that more true than preparing for, or recovering from massive surgery. I didn't have the luxury of getting prepared; mine was emergency surgery. However in her book, *Prepare for Surgery, Heal Faster: A Guide to Mind/Body Medicine,* Peggy Huddleston offers detailed advice on how to take advantage of many helpful modalities before you ever enter the operating room. And it doesn't have to be music as such. There are spoken tapes which encourage an optimistic outlook. There are various CD's available that present sounds of nature for relaxation, such as ocean waves, gentle rain, birdsong, even white noise. In keeping with the principle that what you do with your mind can help your body, in this case to heal, guided imagery exercises (they will be discussed in detail in the next section) can be very helpful. Both Huddleston and Belleruth Naparstek have websites which can open up a whole world of information about relief from the sleeplessness and anxiety which one may feel prior to the Big Day of surgery. Meditation and mindfulness CD's are also available from the *Sounds True* catalogue by such masters a Jon Kabat-Zinn.

Dr. Memet Oz, in *Healing from the Heart*, details how he became convinced that music could be an integral part of preparation and recovery from heart transplant surgery.[67] On a visit to his family in Istanbul, he encountered a noted Turkish healer-scholar-musician named Rahmi Oruc

Guvenc, whose carefully chosen music left Oz and a roomful of relatives and friends feeling relaxed and clear-headed, even as he says, "As if I had imbibed a mind-altering substance.[68] Rahmi, who can be accessed via Google, "explained that sounds based on a five–tone scale affect the limbic system of the brain and emotional changes in listeners can be detected on an EEG, the test that measures brain waves."

When jazz musician Johnny Copeland needed a heart transplant at Columbia Presbyterian Hospital where Oz was developing a Complementary Medicine program, complications left him in a comatose state and near death. Hearing Copeland's "Rainbow Man" on his car radio gave Oz the idea of playing his own music back to him through headphones. It took weeks for him to awaken fully, but six months later, a large contingent of hospital staff attended his first gig at a New York club.

Steven Halpern, PhD, composer, researcher and author of *Sound Healing: the Music and Sounds that Make Us Whole* has produced numerous recordings which are used for healing in schools, hospitals, homes and offices around the world. He points out that sound therapy has been used for a variety of healing purposes since the ancient Greeks.

In *New Choices in Natural Healing* Halpern reminds us that beyond music, we can derive healing from sounds of nature, a walk on the beach, singing to ourselves, playing an instrument, and even learning toning.[69] Having experienced two workshops in this method, which involves what is basically a form of humming, I can attest to its benefits. Directions for this can be found in *New Choices* for what music therapist Don G. Campbell calls, "massaging the body from within."[70]

My toning class was a multi-session experience at a writing conference with Murshida Victoria Angela, a Sufi sound healer, who has done presentations all over the world and at Harvard. We lay in a circle on a carpeted floor in one session and practiced using simple vowel sounds, both short and long, loud and soft, to call forth various feelings, and to assist in healing them. This was six months after my surgery and I found it tiring.

Because of my recent surgery, I became the center of another exercise in healing with sound. Another woman and I were seated in the center of a circle with our backs firmly pressed against each other. Once again, we all hummed our chosen vowel sounds and I could feel the vibration from my partner as well as sense the vibrations of this healing, humming circle.

Once we were warmed up, Victoria asked us to express the deepest angers in our lives with a vowel sound of our own choosing. She walked around our circle, urging us to face what we were really angry about in our lives. I found myself making harsh sounds with the E vowel I had chosen, which at first reminded me of the sounds one makes giving birth. Then I realized what they really were: the sounds I would have made, if conscious, at those who were coming to cut me open–pure animal resistance to being attacked.

Even though my brain/mind was seemingly shut off, my body knew and resented it. After the fact, my intellect knew that the doctors had saved me, but my body was still angry. This helped to explain why I was washed by feelings I felt powerless to resist. It taught me what the feelings were, and over the last five years, I have learned how to manage them.

Dr. Halpern explains that sounds can have an effect on blood pressure, heartbeat, breathing and have been effective in lessening pain in surgical and dental procedures.[71] Music during tests has been shown to affect scores and it surely can improve exercise workouts. I can verify this last item in my Cardiac Rehab exercises. Moving to the beat of some peppy music can make twenty minutes on an elliptical trainer go very quickly.

Limited only by your taste and your ability to surf the internet, there are CD's of singing and chanting from cultures all over the world. Many websites allow for a short sample before you select what works for you. My favorites include a Tibetan musician trained in the ancient art of musical healing, Nawang Khechog; a sound artist called Anugama, and Native American flutist Carlos Nakai. Sound healers Dave and Steve Gordon list twenty possible uses for their "Musical Healing" disc, including childbirth, massage, meals and calming babies, as well as the obvious pre/post-surgical relaxation. Deva Premal is a singer worth exploring, as is Janet Spahr and her unusual instrument, the Hang Drum. Of course each person already has their own favorites. The wonders of modern technology allow you to create your own relaxation playlist.

More than any other aspect about which I am sharing my experiences, music, meditation and sound theory are areas where making selections is very much a matter of personal taste. I tend to prefer a "new age" kind of sound with flutes and bells, but neuroscientist Candace Pert was cheered and energized by her favorite rock music. Indeed, she ends her relaxation

CD with "Let it Shine" by Karen Drucker, a song so upbeat, it gets me dancing around my study.

Gleaned from *New Choices*, I found that Janalea Hoffman, a registered musical therapist, has produced tapes such as "Musical Massage," Musical Acupuncture," and "Musical Hypnosis." A partial list of those Dr. Halpern recommends includes "Seaspace" by Georgia Kelly, "Dolphin Dreams" by Jonathan Goldman, "Inside" by Paul Horn, "Silk Road" by Kitaro and "Spectrum Suite" by Dr. Halpern himself. This last is one I have owned for many years without realizing its healing potential; I am grateful to have a player which can do old cassettes.

All of these can be used in a variety of ways. Peggy Huddleston's book, *Prepare for Surgery, Heal Faster* is worth looking at if you are facing surgery of any kind. Music in your ears is practiced in many hospitals, but you often have to ask for it. In the early stages of recovery soothing sounds can help as you try to relax amid the physical challenges you face and help you to get needed rest. Used at night they can help you off to sleep. Concentrating on the music, the nature sounds or the meditations can provide a welcome distraction from worrying about yourself.

Using some form of healing sound was an adjunct to my daily naps in the early days of my recovery. Now I use certain ones to play softly while I read or write as well. Those that are more specific for total relaxation I still use for naps, but the naps are shorter now, usually only thirty-five to forty minutes. Indeed psychologist Kathy Kastan in *From the Heart: A Woman's Guide to Living with Heart Disease,* strongly suggests not napping for more than an hour.[72] I set a kitchen timer so I can get back to my day feeling refreshed. If your busy life does not settle down until almost bedtime, a specific time set aside to relax can be a helpful prelude to sleep.

For the sake of your continuing health, consider taking time for this important aspect of healing. The research which indicates its many benefits is extensive. Music that makes you feel good as you drive your car can start or end your day more calmly than the horrors of the news, or the stress, not to mention the danger, of your cell phone. Finally, Dr. Halpern advises that whenever possible, "It is a good idea to escape the whirring computers and the growling mowers of everyday life and listen to the sounds of natural silence. Just find a quiet place and take a walk. Your health will be the better for it."[73]

"As gentle and low key as these practices are, they consistently deliver reliable clinical changes, demonstrated by hard-nosed lab values".
Belleruth Naparstek

18

IMAGERY

What is imagery, in a healing context, and how does it work as such a powerful tool? Even in literature "image" is not regarded as mere pictures. It is defined as "sense experience rendered in words." It includes all the senses–taste, touch, smell, sight, hearing, emotions and whole body sensations. Belleruth Naparstek, psychotherapist, author and imagery innovator; one of the recognized authorities on the subject, explains it this way in *Staying Well with Guided Imagery:*

"Guided imagery is a process of deliberately using your imagination to help your mind and body heal, stay well, or perform well. It's a kind of directed daydream, a purposeful creation of positive sensory images in your imagination. For example, you might create images of your immune cells fighting germs, or your pulse slowing down; you might recall in exacting sensory detail an absent loved one for extra emotional comfort; or you could "rehearse" a perfect golf swing moments before you actually heft your club."[74]

In a more clinical discussion in *Everyday Heroes, Survivors of Trauma and How They Heal*, Naparstek describes imagery as "…using words and phrases designed to evoke rich, multisensory fantasy and memory in order to create a deeply immersive, receptive mind-state that is ideal for catalyzing desired changes in mind, body, psyche and spirit. For most people imagery is an easy user-friendly form of meditation that yields immediately felt results. Its gentle nature belies its potency and its research-proven cumulative efficacy…Indeed, given the last twenty years of research findings from various clinical trials, it is surprising that imagery isn't prescribed as a universal, low-cost preventative health tool, much in the way aspirin is used to reduce the likelihood of future heart attacks."[75]

The idea is to relax, focus, and allow your body and mind to "be there.. And yes, the research is there to document its effectiveness in many situations. It has been there for years, as you will see. Naparstek presents a long list of all the conditions for which imagery can be helpful. She ends the list with citing a numbered footnote. Seeking out the citation at the end of the book, one finds one and a third pages of fine print listing the numerous research sources she has reviewed.[76]

Almost everyone uses imagination to help to feel better, but my first experience with specific, focused use of imagery came at, of all places, the luncheon session of a professional conference, of the National Association for Gifted Children. As part of her keynote speech about the power of the mind to influence the body, Barbara Clarke, PhD, of UCLA asked her audience of 400 professionals in the field of gifted studies to stand up. Being by nature an open-minded group, we all did so.

She then asked us to close our eyes, and took us through an exercise where we awakened in a lovely bedroom, opened a door to a lovely California morning, a velvety lawn under our bare feet, and a gorgeous lemon tree. All this was described using great sensory detail. We selected a lemon, felt the surface, sensed its weight in our hands. Then we were directed to pierce the skin with a thumbnail and inhale the lovely scent. We were directed back to our lovely bedroom and awakened.

"If you experienced increased salivation and actually tasted that lemon, please raise your hand," Dr. Clarke requested. Most of the audience did so, including me! "Now look at your hands," she continued. "Anybody have a lemon?" No hands were raised. When a colleague suggested signing up for an imagery workshop being offered in our school district, I registered quickly. When a second course was offered I did the same.

I have made use of my imagery training for others in a variety of situations ever since, especially in writing workshops, to remove writers block and enhance the writer's ability to access their own memories and buried images. Teaching the technique to restless high school students allowed me to offer them a "90-second vacation" where they could image their way to their favorite spot, and release end-of-the-day tensions.

From my own personal use, I can share a few favorites. As a reader you can create your own from my examples, or from the books and tapes of Naparstek. If you are facing a surgical procedure, the work of Peggy Huddleston is also very helpful. Both of these authorities have websites where you can purchase books and tapes.

A sleep image I have used for many years is a beautiful sloping lawn leading down to a small lake with an island in the center. It is a warm sunny day, and the tiny wavelets catch the sunlight and flicker merrily. I try to feel the velvety grass under my bare feet, the sun on my back. I reach the water, look at the pebbles and the mud at the edge of the water and…sleep.

Imagery was also extremely helpful when I had my first attack of diverticulitis, a painful intestinal condition, and several years before my heart surgery. I was given a powerful combination of antibiotics to be taken for 14 days, supposedly the only way to really cure this attack. The result was devastating. I had to cancel teaching at an important writing conference, as well as a trip to help my son and his wife after the birth of their second child.

For a solid week I spent my days flattened in a recliner, nauseous, dizzy, weak and afraid. I would force myself to eat enough to take the pills, which as I perceived them through the amber glass of the pill bottle, appeared to be a bilious shade of green. Distinguishing between the abdominal pain of my condition and the effects of the medication was virtually impossible; I actually feared that I might die. My spiritual beliefs include the concept of Gaia, the Earth Mother. I was at that point, a weeping child, looking for motherly comfort. Through my tears, I imagined her benevolent face above my chair saying, "It's alright, child, you will be alright."

A consult with my gastroenterologist assured me that I would not die, but he urged me to hang in there and complete the 14 days, since I had come this far. The alternative could be another, more severe attack. Sufficiently challenged, and convinced that I did in fact, have to tough this out, I dumped the capsules on my kitchen table and looked at them. They were not green, but a lovely shade of aquamarine, one of my favorite colors.

They became my defenders. Each time the pain and nausea rolled over me, I created an image. They were tall blue goddesses; and each time the ugly bacteria attacked my gut, they fired beams of light which killed the evil invaders. It was fun to watch the battles because the bacteria always lost. It got me through the second week and on to recovery.

The early months of my recovery from the heart surgery illustrate how useful it can be to combine music and imagery to create a space for healing each day. It also illustrates how you can create a place where you can actually go and increase your ability to get well, by taking your mind off yourself for a while. You do this by occupying your mind with the creation of the details of your healing place. Here is how I did it. You will find your own way, and your own time of day, and your own music.

Each afternoon, when I needed a nap anyway, I would go up to my room and get relaxed with a pillow under my knees (it makes a big difference–I strongly recommend it) and a warm cover. The CD I most often used is "Tibetan Meditation Music," by Nawang Khechog, a Tibetan musician trained in the ancient art of healing sound. As the music played, I created the image in great detail. I was in a Tibetan healing monastery, high above a beautiful valley filled with thriving fields and a picturesque village.

The room had been carved out of the mountain and had stone walls, a fireplace, a stone path which ran along the whole side of the mountain, and a soft warm bed. The monks and all the people of the valley, even the children, played musical instruments. There were flutes of all kinds, small bells, echoing horns and small violins.

A little boy would bring firewood, accompanied by a little girl who would sing, and a flute-playing boy. Tall graceful women played deep voiced flutes on the path outside my room. The monks came in and out with music, prayers and chants. I did not need to understand the words. At sunset, deep horns would sound all up and down the valley, gradually fading away as darkness came on. I usually did not hear the end of the CD, as I would be lost in the bliss of a 40 to 50 minute nap.

Another helpful CD was called "Shamanic Dream" by Anugama. Again, a combination of methods was helpful. This CD was one my massage therapist used. I eventually purchased my own because I like it so much. As soon as I hear it, I can image myself getting a massage. I use both CDs for relaxation to this day.

You will use whatever works for you; some people prefer to hear a verbal relaxation tape of the type both Naparstek and Huddleston produce. I encourage you to experiment; exotic locales may fuel your ability to create a relaxing image. The internet offers endless choices, or you may wish to rely on old favorites already in your collection. You don't need to go to a class, hire a therapist, wear special workout clothes, or even leave your house. It's private; it's gentle; it's free, and it works; it is limited only by your own imagination.

"Doll making is a way to free oneself from worries, struggles and emotions. Creating a doll, or any art, directly affects the autonomic nervous system which controls body functions and the immune system."
Barb Kobe, doll maker and teacher.

19

THE ANCIENT ART OF SOUL DOLLS

I first found the Tibetan spirit and bodhisattva known as Green Tara in the Dharma Crafts catalogue filled with beautiful statues more expensive than I could ever afford. I was continuing with a difficult time, many months after coping with four major surgeries—open heart, cataracts, and a colon resection. I was having anxiety attacks, feeling afraid and /or depressed most of the time; wondering if I should just give up on myself and become an aging invalid.

There were several books listed, which I could afford, and I ordered them. When I read that Tara's extended right hand offered compassion and creativity, and her upheld left hand warded off fear, she became my consoler. I especially liked the belief that she was born from the tears of a previous bodhisattva who wept because he couldn't save all beings from suffering. I cut out her picture from the catalogue and tacked it up on the air conditioner above my desk.

Further reading yielded that Tara is famous for offering speedy practical help to anyone who asks, but she is particularly known to dispel fear, and freeing beings from negative states. Venerated by Hindus and Buddhists alike, she is known in Tibet as "She Who Liberates." Her chants are sung by farmers in fields, monks and nuns in monasteries, society ladies in Lhasa and nomads in the vast steppes. (Liner notes *Songs of Tara*, Sounds True, Boulder ,CO, 2011)

Shortly after, there came the International Women's Writing Guild annual conference at Skidmore College, and by coincidence, my resolution that this year, finally, I would take Nina Reimer's Dolls for the Soul Workshop. Nina Ayin Reimer began her career as the medical illustrator of the classic *Our Bodies Ourselves*, in the 1970s. She is a teacher, sculptor, psychic, medical intuitive, Reiki Master, and author of *Artist as Healer: Stories of Transformation and Healing*. (San Francisco, CA: Nina Reimer Publisher, 2003) as well as several children's books.

According to Reimer, dolls have been used across all cultures and many centuries for knowledge and healing. It is an ancient art which can take many forms. Her own dolls are created for private clients using her intuitive gift. As a teacher, she helps others to create their own dolls, which in her workshops come spontaneously to each creator. I had seen the amazing creations shown at each conference, and it seemed that if so many other women could do this, so could I.

We began with an imaging exercise. To the beat of a small quiet drum, paced to match the beating of our own hearts, we closed our eyes and were conducted on a journey. We walked along a lake, crossed a small bridge, and waited on the path for a figure to appear. If no one did, we retraced our steps and accepted that inspiration would come. The idea was that from deep inside our unconscious selves, our hands and our choices would be guided to produce our Soul Doll. As the figure revealed itself, we would gain insights not available in other ways.

As the work began, I had big second thoughts. There were lots of directions to be followed and scariest of all, decisions to be made, creative choices. And I was going to sculpt a Face?! Thanks to Nina's genius for breaking down a complicated process into simple steps, I formed a dowel and some foil into a stand. With pictures and directions for each tiny piece of clay—eyes, nose, cheeks, chin, brows—I actually formed a head and a face, which was baked in a simple microwave oven–no kiln needed. From Nina's collection I selected a pair of paste-on blue eyes, not knowing why I did so.

The emerging face, the blue eyes and my classmates remarking, "She looks like you," reminded me of a dream figure from many years ago. It was actually a nightmare. I was in a jungle setting being pursued by people who wanted to hurt me. I came to a river, and this figure appeared, showed me a boat, and helped me to escape. She was older, had white hair, a soft gentle face and blue eyes. I liked her very much. When I described her to a perceptive friend, the comment was, "That was you! You were saved by your future self." So I chose white hair, actually llama hair supplied by Nina, for her fluffy halo-like hair.

As the other women all around me chose fabric, feathers, jewels, buttons, I lost confidence again. In such a huge collection, what to choose? A lovely shade of light green was my favorite that summer, so I chose a swatch of that for the dress. Eyelet in a matching color turned up, so I took that, still having no idea where I was going.

A third fabric with stripes, in a design that looked Aztec recalled another figure. This one came in an imaging exercise in a class at Skidmore with Native American Mechi Garza. Again it involved a boat, only this time I was back somewhere in time, and I was a young lad in leather sandals, on a mission. I was carrying a suede pouch continuing something very important; I had no idea what. Stepping off the boat onto the clattering wooden slats of the dock, I was met by a very tall figure whose face was not clear. The robe it wore was like the stripes in the fabric box. I sewed it into two long strips, still not knowing why I did it.

Making hands was another chicken-heart moment. Nina helped me with one, which one is quite evident. Needing to speed up my work, I took my doll back to my room to figure out what to do with eyelet and to try to figure out what kind of soul doll was revealing itself to me. That was when it dawned on me that she was Green Tara–a fusion of my deeper self and the wisdom of Tara. When I told Nina who she was, she helped me arrange the hands in the proper position, right hand out in compassion and creativity, left hand up to ward off fear. At last I felt like I knew where I was going.

In the endless boxes of decorations I, the heart patient, found a heart shaped crocheted piece about two inches wide and placed over Tara's heart. Next a circular piece of glass fitted over that. Adding color to the face was tricky, but again, Nina had a way that even I could manage. The Aztec stripes were wrapped around her neck and draped to form an inverted V down the back. Gold buttons turned up, and heart shaped seashells. The buttons were added to the eyelet on the sleeves and the seashells adorned the Aztec stripes.

Nina's final action is to take the doll out of the room, and see what it tells her. To me she said, "Tara can teach you a lot, but you know a lot too, and you must teach it to others. (At that time I had no idea I would write this book) Also, she would like to have an image of Green Tara to hold."

The following weekend, at a celebration of my birthday, Tara was unveiled to comments of, "Wow! You made that?"

"She looks like a bishop," my nine-year-old granddaughter opined.

Back home, I considered scanning the image I had first found in the Dharma Crafts catalogue and gluing it to the pink stone over her heart, but it proved too difficult to make it so small. I added some small Swarofski crystals to her sleeves, but how to give her the figure that Nina said she had asked for? And how to translate her mantra *Om tare Tuttare Ture Soha?*

Dharma Crafts came through again with a tiny medallion of Tara carved in green stone, mounted on sterling silver, with a silver chain. All I had to do was double the chain and it fit perfectly. The pink glass had to go, but it was worth it—and the $45 I spent. Not to be outdone in being good to myself, I also acquired a sterling Mobius strip with Tara's mantra, which I enjoy wearing when I need to have confidence.

Seeking to translate the mantra, I found help from an Indian doctor, an acquaintance who is a devout Hindu. She provided me with a website featuring one of the many translations according to the Tibetan tradition. (YouTube, Green Tara Mantra, 108 repetitions)

OM—Tara's sacred body and mind;

Tare—Liberation from all discontent;

Tuttare—Liberation from the eight fears, external dangers, but mainly from delusions;

Ture—Liberation from duality, cessation of confusion;

Soha—May the meaning of the mantra take root in my mind.

The details on the site provided enough inspiration for a lifetime. It also featured a beautiful melody for the 108 repetitions to soothe when troubled, or when sending healing energy to another person who may be suffering. Visually it shows a collage of images to go with the singing. It also has other links to chanting sites which added to my knowledge.

My reading books about Tara yielded another version of her origin which I find appealing. She was, as are many figures in Indian mythology, a princess, who with great compassion for suffering, spent her life doing good works. To achieve her goal of reincarnation as a bodhisattva, the court advisors told her to pray to be incarnated as a man. Her reply was that there were already enough male bodhisattvas; she would be the first female. She vowed to always be reborn in female form to serve the needs of women seeking enlightenment.

But there was more to come. My sister Kathleen is the source of wonderful presents at birthdays and Christmas. Last year I opened my holiday gift to find a beautifully detailed copper Tara. I placed her on the bookshelf near my desk, but she needed a properly colorful Indian setting. A brightly colored fabric with many yellows, reds and oranges did the trick. I had purchased this remnant many years ago because I found it lovely, and it had wandered around the house without a use.

Now it is a perfect backdrop for my Friend—for that is what she has become. She pushes away fears and offers compassion—and reminds me to offer it to others. In copper form in my study; in her Soul Doll form on my bedroom bureau, she is a presence in my life. Reciting her mantra is an excellent way to lull me to sleep. Like another benevolent goddess of the West, she comes, "Speaking words of wisdom, let it be, let it be."

> *"Blood pressure can be reduced by stroking a stuffed animal."*
> Nischala Joy Devi in *The Healing Path of Yoga*

20

TITUS AND ME

So here, nine years out, should a mature lady still have a stuffed bear, with whom she sleeps every night? Absolutely! Somewhere in the fog of the early days in the ICU, I demanded, "What happened to the bear?" referring, of course, to the small brown bear given to me by Chuckles the Clown. "I think it's in the closet with your clothes," my husband replied, and out he came.

Placed on my bedside table, "Livey" became the subject of jokes by my surgeon: "Who is this fellow?" He had his vital signs taken along with mine by the physician's assistant, and generally was made much of by the staff. Most of all, I felt comforted by his presence, a welcome distraction from the multiple miseries and discomforts of the post-surgical experience.

In the confusion of my first days at home, someone took the small bear and sat him between the pillows on our bed. He has been there ever since. I reminded my husband, who was amused by his presence, that his name was Live-y. Being of a scholarly bent, he replied that Livy was a Roman historian, and the next day looked up his full name: Titus Livius. In keeping with his belief that this little stuffed creature with the stitched brown eyes and the checkered necktie was a factor in getting me through those first dicey days in the ICU, Tom awarded him the title, "Titus Livius, Ursus Medicus"—Titus, for short.

Why is he still here? Two reasons: One is that we have always been amused by "Stuffies," as are many adults, not all residing in nursing homes. A friend who is extremely talented in sewing once undertook to make stuffed animals of all sizes and shapes. She created everything from piglets dressed as ballerinas to bears the size of a small child. She sold over 50 of them, mostly for adults. I have several friends, professional women, who never travel without a favorite stuffie.

Our current menagerie consists of a Dalmatian, a gift from our oldest daughter; his incredibly real appearance sometimes shocks visitors to our living room. Our front hall is guarded by D.B. Platypus, a dignified and solemn sort, and Pierre the Bear, the K-Mart bear of Christmas, 2000. He is the only one with a wardrobe; it covers up his Christmas shirt in other seasons.

My poetry workshop sent a small unicorn while I was recovering from the surgery, and a friend sent a tiny white bear—with wings. Both wound up on the bookshelf in Tom's study and were named Ulysses and Bianca as he adopted them. "Ulysses laughs at me. He keeps me honest," he insists. We are simply of the persuasion that all things are animate. We talk to the deer that cross the back of our acre, the squirrels, the birds, the trees, the plants. Happily mad? We may be, but it helps to keep us cheerful.

The second reason for Titus' abiding presence is his function as my Rogerian therapist, that being the kind of therapist who just feeds you back your own statements, which helps you to figure things out for yourself. That Titus is both silent and appears wise is a big advantage. When I tell him my troubles, he offers no advice. I can confide all my silly whining to him in complete confidence. I am left to work things out for myself. When I travel, he comes along if it is more than a night or two. A hug from him is a big help in easing the fears that still arise with any strange ache or pain when I am far from home.

As I have said elsewhere, you never get rid of the scary—you just learn to manage it. Titus is my Assistant Manager.

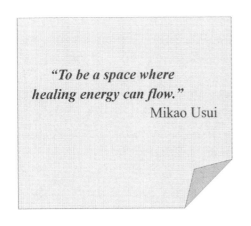

"To be a space where healing energy can flow."
Mikao Usui

21

REIKI

My most recent modality to explore has been Reiki, a hands-on energy therapy which, though still controversial in some areas, is gaining increasing acceptance in the medical profession. What does Reiki do? How does it work? Only the first question has an answer.

Reiki balances the energy field by the simple practice of the laying on of the hands at specific points on the body, these having been "attuned" by a master teacher. The second question must await more sophisticated measurements of what is called the biofield–the energy field which surrounds us all, and which is slowly yielding to scientific investigation. I approached my study of this form with my usual research question: Does this stuff work?

During the first phase of my cardiac rehab at the hospital, the subject came up, and one of the physical therapists shared a story. They had an open heart surgery patient who had a friend come in and give her a Reiki treatment every day, starting the day after her surgery. According to the therapist, there was a noticeable difference in her rate of recovery, and she went home a day earlier than expected.

My first personal experience with Reiki came when it was offered as part of a massage by Mary Ellen; it is often combined with other modalities in this way. The peace and relaxation that resulted was very impressive. I said later that I felt as though I was floating several inches above the surface of the massage table, and I resolved to find out more about it.

First, I read a book, *Reiki, A Comprehensive Guide,* by Josephine Miles.

A practitioner and Reiki Master for 35 years, Miles gives a complete overview of the history, practice, research, acceptance and usefulness of Reiki. She has developed Reiki programs in major hospitals and cites, programs where Reiki is used in institutions from Maine to California, and for a wide variety of diseases and aliments; and during surgery and to ease patients into anesthesia. According to Miles, research validating Reiki is scattered across various medical specialties, but it does exist. The book proved to be a comprehensive resource with diagrams for self-treatment and advice for finding reputable practitioners and teachers.

The value of touch has been an integral part of the healing arts for centuries. Reiki is simply one of the most recent manifestations of that art. Originating in Japan in the early twentieth century, Reiki was developed by Mikao Usui (1865-1926) a householder who was self-educated in spiritual practices, medicine and healing. During a solitary meditation in a mountain retreat, he experienced a profound awakening to the universal energy which surrounds us. He later realized that the careful placing of his hands could transmit that energy in a healing way to others.

Teaching this technique to a Dr. Hayashi (1900-1980) they established a center in Japan. Another of Usui's chief students was Hawayo Takata, and she eventually brought the practice to North America. Reiki Master Teachers designate themselves by their "lineage," that is, how many Masters between them and the Usui school. Thus, a teacher may say that he or she is a sixth generation teacher in the Usui tradition, and name the five teachers which are the connection back to Usui himself. The wide variety of approaches found all over the world today all stem from these three original teachers.

There are three stages of Reiki courses: Reiki I, Reiki II, and Master Class. A fourth level is Master Teacher which must be taught by another Master teacher. As with any tradition passed down, there have been many variations developed. Another book which proved helpful is *Self-Healing with Reiki,* by British energy healer Penelope Quest. She outlines these levels as follows. Level I is where you receive "attunements" to open up your inner healing channels and allow the Reiki energy to flow through you. The emphasis here is on giving yourself a treatment as well as others.

Reiki II includes more attunements, drawing sacred symbols that come from ancient Sanskrit, and learning to use them with Reiki. It provides greater scope for personal healing and spiritual development. One may also learn a form of distant healing, and this level usually requires a two day workshop.

Level III is that of Master Teacher where you will learn how to perform attunements so that you can teach others. It can involve becoming an apprentice to a Master for a period of up to a year. Unlike the first two levels, this one means making a lifelong commitment. According to Quest, it can be a very demanding but very rewarding journey.

I decided to study with a chiropractor and healer in my own area, Master Teacher Dr. Lauren Nappen. Her teaching has come down in a direct line from Usui, Hayashi, and Tanaka in seven steps. The course I took was Reiki I. I offer my experience as evidence that it is a helpful healing method which can be used on others, but most importantly, on yourself.

On a sunny Saturday morning, six students gathered around a table in a windowed healing space filled with light for our first session: a musician, myself, a woman caring for a husband with dementia; a veterinarian, a person already trained in Reiki, and a woman dealing with anxiety issues.

A brief booklet filled us in on the history of Reiki, included photos of Usui, and explained its basic principle, to be a space through which healing energy can flow. Reiki involves a rather simple exchange of energy; energy that is readily available all around us in the universe. Properly directed it can offer healing. You are not expected to DO anything, our teacher explained. Properly attuned, you will simply allow your hands to channel healing energy where it needs to go.

Dr. Lauren then demonstrated the various hand positions on herself. They were also illustrated in our booklets. After this, we were invited to sit quietly, breathe gently, and prepare ourselves for attunement. One by one we were called into an adjacent room. Music played softly as we waited.

And here, of course, is where my natural skepticism kicked in. We were counseled to pay attention to what we felt during the attunement: heat, pressure or anything else. I was in "Does this stuff work?" mode as Dr. Lauren greeted me with a smile and asked me to sit down, close my eyes, and rest my hands, palms up, on my thighs.

Attunements are at the core of Reiki practice. They help us to focus the energy as a clearer channel. Dr. Lauren moved her hands around a short distance from my upper body. This is Attunement I is giving access to the heart and our feeling life. Next, she moved her hands around my throat and shoulders, for Attunement II, our ability to communicate. Last, she placed her hands on top of my head, our place of higher consciousness, feeling well and alive. As this proceeded, I began to feel a very strong pressure in the centers of my upturned palms, and I silently observed, "She is nowhere near my hands."

A digression is needed here.

Several months before, I had been involved in an energy "game" in a class with a Tai Chi teacher at the annual conference of the International Women's Writing Guild. As luck would have it, my partner was a highly experienced yoga instructor, and Reiki Master Teacher, Yael Flusberg of Washington, D.C. To begin, we were directed to extend our hands, one with palms up, the other above, with palms down. The object was to see if we could feel the energy force between us. With five or six inches between our palms, we started to feel a very strong pressure-like force. Our eyes met, and we began to giggle, taking turns with palms top and bottom, playing with a very real force.

On her website, Yael describes Reiki this way. "It is a gentle hands-on healing art that jump-starts the body's self-healing mechanisms. At this physical level, Reiki is particularly good at balancing the autonomic nervous system, which regulates over 90 percent of your internal functions, including hormonal and immune system responses, digestion and sleep. At the emotional level, Reiki helps to create a state of peacefulness and as such is great for safely exploring a wide range of personal issues."

What I felt on my open palms during the attunement with Dr. Lauren was the same force. Conclusion: this stuff is real. Back in the group, some reported pressure, some heat; one said she got very cold. We divided into two groups of three. I drew the musician and the vet, a lucky choice. Practicing the proper placement of hands (with coaching) we gave and received a full-body Reiki treatment lasting about 45 minutes each.

While the receiving was as restful as a good massage, it was the giving that provided, to me, the most powerful evidence that this is a useful modality. Placing my hands on certain parts of my fellow student's bodies, my hands became so heavy that I almost felt that I would not be able to move them if I tried. Our teacher explained that this is a manifestation of the energy going where it needs to go, and you should just allow yourself to be a channel. There is no ego involved.

For all the importance of sharing, both our teacher, Josephine Miles and, of course, Penelope Quest agree, that the most important use of this healing energy is on yourself. Our commitment was to use it in this way for 21 days and then attend a short follow-up class. Several classmates reported easing of anxieties, the wife reported a small breakthrough with her husband, and the vet was amazed at its effect on two aging dogs with joint issues. I used it at bedtime and found it eased my whirling daytime mind and helped me off to sleep very regularly. It also helps to ease indigestion, I found, and my arthritic knee when it acts up. Placing my hands on the back of a friend who was fighting cancer, he reported that he could feel a healing force. I plan on taking Reiki II when next it is offered. With more skill I can help both myself and others.

For the skeptics, Penelope Quest offers this quote from Hippocrates in the fifth century BC:

"It is believed by experienced doctors that the heat which oozes out of the hand, on being applied to the sick, is highly salutary. It has often appeared, while I have been soothing my patients, as if there was a singular property in my hands, to pull and draw away from the affected parts aches and diverse impurities by laying my hand upon the place and extending my fingers toward it. Thus it is known to some of the learned that health may be implanted in the sick by certain gestures and by contact, just as some diseases may be communicated from one to another."[77]

Most teachers seem to agree that unless you wish to become a teacher or a practitioner, the most important reason for studying Reiki is to use it on yourself. The thinking is that as you become more balanced and peaceful yourself, you will have more to offer to others. This is not limited to a treatment you may be able to give to a needy friend, but to your whole approach to relating to the world as a peaceful and balanced human being.

> *"It's not about your back.
> It's about your entire nervous
> system. It's about your life."*
> Lauren Nappen, DC

21

CHIROPRACTIC

As I prepared this book I did not intend to cover chiropractic as a healing modality, since I had not made use of it in my healing journey. A massive back spasm, an agonizing expansion of my ongoing right shoulder trapezius problem, changed all that. As in the past, my conventional primary doctor, over-busy and over the phone, offered me pain killers and a muscle relaxant as the only approach. Of course, the pills provided some initial relief. But if the pain was as agonizing as I described, I was instructed to go to the ER for x-rays. Experienced by now in caring for myself, and wondering what x-rays could do to look at muscle, I chose to ignore the advice about the ER.

I called my massage therapist, who agreed to see me the next day and worked on the affected area only very gently. We agreed that more work was needed. The healer with whom I had studied Reiki has been a practitioner of what she calls "gentle chiropractic" for over twenty years. A phone call yielded a receptionist who said, "Oh muscles spasms! I have them too; aren't they awful?" there followed several minutes of cheery commiseration, which began, even then, to ease my pain.

An initial consultation with Dr. Lauren Nappen at her healing center, *Ahhhjusting to Life*, gave me insight into this healing method well beyond the manipulation of one's backbone. First, I filled out a detailed medical history, and a questionnaire about how I viewed various aspects of my current life, and answered questions about lifestyle and life events. It was introduced in the following way:

These pages of questions offer me a glimpse into your life story. The same places, faces and events that have fashioned and molded your life have also created the circumstances that have led you to this place and time of concern...In understanding your biography, your biology comes into greater focus.

Then Dr. Lauren took out her model of the human spine and explained the basics of how it works. Like many people, I was vaguely aware of vertebrae and the discs which cushion them, allowing flexibility in the spine and bony protection for the spinal cord. What I was not aware of, was the openings on the side of each vertebrae through which pass the nerve fibers which connect the brain to the entire body—muscles, bones, organs, fingers, toes, digestion, respiration, heart function, etc., etc.

As Dr. Lauren explained, "It's not about your back; it's about your entire nervous system, which is in touch with every part of you– consciousness to neurotransmitters, to neuropeptides, to synapses, to nerve cells and fibers, to nerve pathways, nerve roots, to spinal cord and your brain–one huge network of communication!" Tall and slender, her dark hair close cropped, she leans back in her chair, her eyes wide with merry smiling.

She explained further that events in life, physical, chemical or emotional, can interfere with this wonderful network, and are usually the result of what are called vertebral subluxations.

These are the stretching, twisting or irritation of the spinal cord and its associated nerve roots that compromise the conversation that your body is having with itself to maintain health and well being. Chiropractic seeks to locate and reduce this nerve system interference. An interesting new idea— I never quite thought of my body as having a conversation with itself.

Next, there was a detailed physical exam of me lying on an examining table, sitting, and standing, while she made notes on a diagram of the spine from front and side angles. Over the fourteen years since the original injury, I had nerve block injections from a neurologist, trigger point massage from my excellent massage therapist, ice, heat—but the spasms always repeated themselves eventually. This examination revealed imbalances in the areas of my upper cervical spine directly connected to the areas of difficulty with my right shoulder and upper back. Her theory: the imbalance occurred with the original injury, and the "glitch" in my spinal column was compensated for, but was never really resolved; thus the repetition of the spasms.

If I had been directed to a massage therapist and/or a chiropractor fourteen years ago, could much of this have been avoided? I was reminded of my experience with the heart symptoms. If I had been made aware of what I only discovered five months *after* my surgery, could I have avoided eighteen months of misdiagnosis , anxiety and further damage to my heart? Once again, my experience illustrates the need for conventional and integrative medicine to join forces to accomplish true long-lasting healing for the patient.

Dr. Lauren agrees. "It's convenient and controllable for the health care system to define chiropractic as only about your back. That's where the authorities miss out on the fact that others may know something about living and dying, and the quality of life in between."

An adjustment in this form of gentle chiropractic proceeds like this. I lie face down on a narrow padded table, head in a face-hole, folded arms resting below the table on a cushion, giving the table a hug. Time passes— time for the spine to settle into position. Next, gentle hand pressure is applied, in my case, to the upper back/spine and the lower back. This happens a number of times, with waiting in between. A small device which snaps a short pulse against my neck is used. Dr. Lauren has named it "Rosie the Riveter." It does not hurt.

I roll over on my back and Dr. Lauren sits at the head of the table and cradles my head. More specific pressures are exerted on certain areas of my neck and shoulders; more use of Rosie, but gently. Then I am finished for the day. I completed a twelve-week program of gently re-aligning my upper spine and certain areas of my lower back, bit by bit. Does this stuff work? It seems to. As I continue to have regular adjustments, not only my back will stay aligned, but the energy which travels along my spine will remain balanced.

But how and why does all this happen? The same old question is asked of this healing method as all the others. "Where is the research?" Dr. Lauren sighs. "Someone's experience outweighs the research any time," in her opinion. "You can get too far into the science and then you lose your innate knowing, but you can lose balance on either side."

Dr. Lauren admits that she sometimes grows weary of explaining how much cutting-edge, Twenty-first Century research supports the basic premises of chiropractic care. She gives me a quick history lesson and several up to date sources.

Although various touch therapies have been utilized by healers in all cultures for thousands of years, what we think of as chiropractic (from the Greek, 'done with the hand') appeared around 1895 with the work of Dr. D.D. Palmer, a magnetic healer, and later his son. They were always looking for the how and why of the body, never to make disease go away. The founding principle of chiropractic is that illness is somehow a breakdown in the body's system of communication described earlier.

According to R.W. Stephenson's *The Chiropractic Textbook* of 1927, each living thing has an inborn intelligence, called Innate Intelligence, and the forces of this intelligence operate through the nervous system. Interference with the transmission of these forces can be the cause of disease. This interference is almost always directly or indirectly due to subluxation of the spinal column.

It has taken a long time for these ideas to be accepted as legitimate. In the 1920s chiropractors were jailed for practicing medicine without a license, while their patients were getting well. In contrast to today, Lauren Nappen's doctorate from the College of Straight Chiropractic is recognized; she is licensed by the state, and Medicare covers my adjustment.

Underpinning the work of modern chiropractic, is research in the rarest levels of cellular biology and neurobiology. For explanations Dr. Lauren recommends, among others, the work of Bruce Lipton, cellular biologist, the late Candace Pert, and Dr. Donald Epstein, developer of Network Spinal analysis. The latter is the method in which Dr. Lauren is trained, and hence the gentle touches I have received.

Lipton's work over twenty years has caused him to conclude, as the earlier chiropractors did, that each of the 50 trillion cells in the human body has its own intelligent life. On a practical basis, he says that our thoughts release chemistry, and our cells are bathed in whatever chemistry the brain sends out—positive or otherwise. Not feeling well? Lipton recommends that as you prepare for a visit to a conventional doctor, ask yourself what might be going on in your life to cause you to feel so badly. He believes that most illness comes from unconscious beliefs, which if made conscious, can be utilized for healing.

According to Caroline Myss in *Anatomy of the Spirit* "As

neurobiologist Dr. Candace Pert has proven, neuropeptides—the chemicals triggered by emotions—are thoughts converted into matter. Our emotions reside physically in our bodies and interact with our cells and tissues…through a highly complex process."[78]

Pert herself, in best-selling *Molecules of Emotion* describes, "A new breed of chiropractors who differ from the conventional ones in that they bring an awareness of energetic, emotional levels to their healing."[79] Enter Dr. Donald Epstein, founder of Network Spinal Analysis Chiropractic, who treated Dr. Pert and in whose method Dr. Lauren is trained.

In an interview in *Positive Health Magazine, "Allowing a Higher Level of Human Function,"* by Jenny Thomas (June 2005), Epstein says," I found that by using gentle and specific touches in a consistent sequence, where the spinal cord attaches to the spine, a patient's own body learns to release complex patterns of tension and areas of disablement."

It occurs to me now that even after all this time, I may have more work to do on myself, and that chiropractic may be an important avenue to pursue. This is true especially in light of Dr. Pert's statement that "…trauma and blockage of emotional and physical information can be stored indefinitely at cellular level."[80]

Taking all this together, chiropractic makes wonderful sense. If emotions, stress and trauma, etc., can cause negative effects on our physical body, more positive beliefs can help us to heal from them. But just as important, is that working correctly on crucial areas of the physical body can work this grand communication network, this conversation that the body is having with itself, in the other direction, and heal our emotions as well.

Dr. Lauren smiles as she says, "The culture is on the verge of shifting; it may take a few more hundred years."

> *"This is your world; it is your feast…Look at the greatness of the whole thing. Look, don't hesitate—look! Open your eyes. Don't blink, and look, look—look further."*
> Chogyam Trungpa

22

GARDENING AS MEDITATION

Like yoga, meditation is often equated with an image of an exotic figure seated cross-legged, eyes closed, and seemingly in a trance-like state. And like yoga, this is one form it may take, but there are many other forms. In contemporary society things are simpler.

Meditation is a healing practice accessible to anyone, and can be practiced almost anywhere. In its many variations, it seems ideally suited for people with busy over-scheduled lives. It is as easy as taking a few minutes several times a day, to sit quietly, close your eyes, breathe gently but deeply, and simply be in the moment, aware of your true self and what is really going on in your mind. It can be done in the morning as you arise, on the bus or train going to work, having a quiet solitary lunch, sitting at your desk, or recovering from an aggravating session with your boss.

In *YOU, Staying Young* Dr. Oz says, "In a world with more noise than a pre-school classroom, our brains (and souls) need moments of silence to recharge, refocus and become rejuvenated."[81] Most of the authors I consulted agreed that regular practice of some form of meditation creates a measureable relaxation response which can result in lowering of blood pressure, relief of chronic pain, easing of muscle tension, diminishing of anger and frustration, and lowering of stress hormones such as the now familiar cortisol.

In *New Choices in Natural Healing*, Dr. Joan Borysenko says, "Everybody gets into a state of meditation several times a day without really calling it that." (Or realizing its value?) "It could have been when digging in the garden, playing with a child, or watching a sunset. For that moment, past and future faded away and you were living in the present moment. That's a form of meditation."[82]

The most notable person associated with mindfulness and meditation is John Kabat-Zinn of the University of Massachusetts Hospital's Stress Reduction Clinic, known worldwide for his work in the use of mindfulness meditation as a healing modality. In Bill Moyers' *Healing and the Mind,* he describes it this way: "Meditation just has to do with paying attention in a particular way.[83] There is no agenda, no place to go, nothing to do. Just be here, hanging out with yourself."[84]

For me, hanging out with myself means spending time with an oval of grass, trees and bushes behind my house, which I am pleased to call a Zen garden. My Zen garden is something I have worked on since 1980. It is a 15 by 20 oval in the back of our acre, aligned with the sunrise and sunset of March. That is when I began, with two rocks who "liked each other." Then came dark brick stones at the sunset end and white stones at sunrise. Over the years there have been lots of trials, some wonderful mistakes, and much learning for me.

Early on, I said to one of my students, "I have absolutely no idea what I am doing here."

"I do," she replied. "You are drawing the mandala of your soul in the earth."

I like that idea. It has seemed over the years that when I am a mess, so is the garden. Fixing it up helps to straighten me out. Sitting amidst the stones picking weeds, the world goes away. It is often the best method for solving a problem, or discovering that the problem is not nearly as earthshaking as I thought. Observing some of the tiniest aspects of nature leads to philosophical insights that continually surprise me. I now understand why Zen monks spend so much time raking the stones in their gardens.

Many lessons are to be learned here. Gone are the days when I could plant 120 annuals in an afternoon, and drench the garden in color. Now, I can work for an hour or so, and must plan my chores accordingly, and accept with grace the limitations that I live with. One day, as I ran out of energy, I was tempted to despair and give up gardening altogether, when the

Little Voice reminded me of a quote from the poet Rumi, which applies to a lot more than gardening: "If all you can do is crawl…start crawling."

Today I am enjoying the late afternoon of a glorious cloud-splashed day—a gift that August sometimes gives us. It is 80 degrees, a breeze, birds twittering in the maples and evergreens, completely without the help of electronics. The grass has blossomed in to a field of clover, so I am watching the bees enjoying themselves

I have tried to stay non-representational in the garden, so the white stones focus on the two rocks who liked each other, and a gnarled piece of a lightning-struck tree to remind me that life is full of unexpected events. The dark stones once had a piece of driftwood that reminded me of the silhouette of a Japanese sage, but it slowly rotted away (another lesson) and is now a small decoration. Presently there is the stump of a tree, upended so the roots form a free-form sculpture. It was pulled up when we had the front walk rebuilt, and tossed aside by the workmen. I enjoyed the looks I got when I gleefully carted it away like some great treasure.

The dark stones and the white stones are now linked by two foot-wide beds of flowers, trees and bushes, thus forming the oval. There is a bench, but I don't use it much for meditation. As I have finally learned, the work of keeping this garden IS meditation. I have concluded that reaping the rewards of meditation means finding your own garden, wherever in your life it exists.

23

THE LESSONS
WHAT DID I LEARN?

I am by nature a curious problem-solver, by profession a writer, and a sometime nosy journalist. Most of what I learned, I figured out for myself by observing what was happening in my own body. Then I found it verified in my own research. I asked myself over and over, "What is happening to me? What causes this? Am I going crazy? How can I deal with these symptoms? What can account for these waves of depression/anxiety which appear out of nowhere and wash over me in waves for no apparent reason? Why do I constantly put a fear/negativity interpretation on the simplest situations? Why do I sometimes enter the kitchen for breakfast and when my husband says good morning, I burst into tears? Will I have to live with this psychological pain for the rest of my life? Are the medications doing more harm than good? I know about yoga and massage, but do any of these other healing modalities work? These were just a few of the questions I asked, over a period of several years.

One of the things I learned is that there is a difference in the post-event experience of those who have had what we call a "heart attack," and the kind of cardiac train wreck some of us experience. The heart malfunctions. Treatment is given in the form of meds, rest, possible intervention with a stent—a mild intervention, no more traumatic than some tests.

The patient recovers without needing a major invasion of the body. These are the people who usually move on with their lives, and can truly "forget about it," over time. If they can make the proper lifestyle changes,

154

they may never have a reoccurrence. Such patients could be the ones who prompted a statement to me by a hospital administrator that, "Most people I know who have a heart attack forget about it and go on with their lives."

Not so for those of us whose experience involves a major breakdown of the heart's function. These damages to the heart or arteries require actual physical repair or even removal and replacement of parts of the cardio-vascular equipment.

This will usually involve a major invasion of the body cavities, notably the chest, as well as the "harvesting" of veins from legs or other areas in bypass surgery. The sternum (breastbone) is opened with a bone saw. The heart itself, and/or the adjacent arteries are actually physically handled, and parts sometimes repaired or replaced with manmade pieces. The patient is kept alive on a heart-lung machine while all this takes place. This is notable in the repair and replacement of heart valves and the bypassing of multiple arteries.

Many systems must be activated to ensure that the patient can survive this dual assault on the body, both from the heart's problems and the trauma of the operation. The chief of these is the bypass, or heart-lung machine, which stands in for the patient's organs while the heart is being repaired. Anesthesia must be employed so that the patient is not conscious of what is being done to them. Blood supply to the unconscious brain must be carefully calibrated so as not to leave the patient with a repaired heart but a damaged brain. More recently, techniques have been developed to operate without the use of the heart-lung machine.

Re-starting the heart when the procedure is completed is another challenge. If the electrical spark does not "catch," the patient will die on the table. Tending wounds, preventing infection, re-establishing completely disarranged bodily functions and body chemistry, chest drains to prevent dangerous accumulation of fluids, catheter to monitor kidney function, resuming nutrition and elimination; pain control for all of the above, are all processes which must be regulated with pacemakers, pills, drains, IVs, etc.

These procedures, though necessary to save the patient's life, are in themselves a horrendous assault upon the person's body. They cause damage which must then be repaired along with the cardiac symptoms. What happens to the body happens to the mind and spirit? Therein lies the challenge to the process of true healing, and to the practitioners of contemporary medicine, whether allopathic or integrative.

I see the situation this way: At the center of focus today are the miraculous things medical science and surgery are able to do to save lives—valve replacements, stents, pacemakers, even artificial hearts and human heart replacements. But on either side are, in my opinion, diverse unresolved issues.

On one side is the prevention and detection of heart disease, especially in women, which *should* be saving more lives than it is currently. The miracles cannot be performed if women are sent home instead to the hospital. On the other side is the slow progress of opening medical minds to the full panoply of healing methods, some thousands of years old, which *could* be saving more lives than they are currently doing.

The newest thinking has finally identified effects of massive surgery on the body as having the same potential for long-term negative effects as bombs, plane crashes, earthquakes, assaults, wars, and other disasters. The body, though unconscious, remembers the event on a very deep level. It is now recognized that the same symptoms, which are referred to as PTSD— Post Traumatic Stress Disorder–can be felt by patients after massive surgical procedures. Some rare doctors/therapists offer recognition and treatment.

How could I not only recover, which my doctors assured me I was doing, and rehab, which I worked at diligently, but how could I heal myself and get my life back? I understood that my days of day-long gardening and large home improvement projects were over. Getting my life back meant to me, a feeling that mind and body, for all the limitations, had fused with my soul and spirit to heal me on mitochondrial and chakra levels. After years on my journey, I feel that I am almost there. Another quote from Bellaruth Naparstek in *Invisible Heroes* points toward a better future. "Survivors who fared best were those who researched their own options, found out about new therapies, tried various combinations and essentially took charge of their own healing."[85]

The biggest thing I learned is this. You are the ultimate healer—not the nurses, not the surgeons, the doctors, the cardiologists; not the pharmacist, not the physical therapist. All of them are the facilitators, those who repair what has gone wrong, and/or assist you in the management of the actions you need to take, or refrain from, to manage the rehabilitation and recovery of your body and mind. You need them to assist you as you re-integrate and re-balance the energy forces which you alone can manage, to become whole and sound again.

What you do with your body can heal, or not heal, your mind; and what you do with your mind, can heal, or not heal, your body. The integration of body, mind, soul and spirit constitutes true healing.

24

WHAT I SHOULD HAVE SAID—
WHAT THE DOCTOR SHOULD HAVE SAID

Recall, if you will the earlier scene when a cardiologist wanted to put me on tranquilizers for mild anxiety and depression. Eight and a half years later, knowing what my body and my research have taught me, this is what I should have said.

"Excuse me doctor, for contradicting those with years of education and expertise, but that is the wrong answer. Here is what you should have said:

"Yes, Marylou, I'm afraid the anxiety and depression kind of come with the territory in a situation like yours, and you were wise to let us know. The research shows that these feelings can be triggered by a hormone in your body called cortisol. It is your fight or flight substance, built in from our earliest evolutionary times, activated when you are in any kind of danger. It floods your body with the chemicals you need to survive whether it is an earthquake, an assault, a plane crash, a bomb, combat in war—or the massive surgery which you have experienced.

Although the surgery saved your life, it was a terrific assault on all the systems of your body, mind and spirit. Now, intellectually you know all this. But down on cellular level, your mitochondria (the basic energy cells of your body) only know that you have been attacked.

These chemical triggers can remain on high alert for up to a year, or even longer, if you have new stressful events in your life. The least little thing can set them off, even though it seems that you have pretty well recovered from the actual operation. So the first thing you can do for yourself is to understand that this is body chemistry, that it needs time to settle down, and that each time it happens, it will pass.

We could put you on some sort of tranquilizer right away, but that has its own set of problems and side effects. There is a whole selection of other healing modalities that you can use to help you toward more tranquility. They are often called integrative medicine because they come from traditions other than Western medicine. Using them can put you in charge of your own healing. Although as doctors and surgeons modern medicine allows us to repair your body when things go wrong, true healing must come from within the patient over time.

You have probably heard of some of these methods. They include massage, mindfulness tapes, Reiki, yoga, relaxation and imaging exercises, music and other forms of sound therapy (a new and growing field) aromatherapy, Tai Chi, and the support of others who have "been there done that." You can make contact which such people by following up faithfully with all the phases of your Cardiac Rehab program.

Here is a short pamphlet called "Living Your Best Life After a Cardiac Event." It explains briefly what each of the items I mentioned might be able to do for you. It gives pointers about locating materials and certified practitioners.

We are now affiliated with a cardiac psychologist to whom we can refer you, and we are recommending that you set up an appointment with her for a single consultation about what to expect as you deal with the emotional after-effects of the surgery. It your depression and anxiety worsens, you can seek more regular sessions with our therapist. And there is always prescription relief if you feel it is necessary. Trying some of these methods can heal rather than medicate, and that is what we all want to happen. Good luck."

That is what doctors should be able to say to their patients. And someone should write that pamphlet. While we are waiting, I hope that this little book may be of use. And so I move through the eighth year of my new life. My son Tom calls me each December 8th, and wishes me Happy Birthday. Hey, if I'm only eight, I should be able to get away with a lot. Two final poems express my feelings as I look ahead, and my appreciation of a spouse who has stood by me through it all.

GARDEN WITHOUT OAKS

For Tom

Two willows lean together,
bending low in storms,
rising together when they pass,
determined not to fall
and leave just one
standing alone.

THE ROAD

For Alice Orr

Dorothy's faith in the future allowed her
that foot-crossing skippy-step down
the yellow brick road to the Wizard,
arm in arm with her friends, a lion
a tin man, a stumbling scarecrow.

There we were, Alice and me walking
up a hill, circling the building to find
an elevator, climbing away from our
train wrecks–her double mastectomy,
my rebuilt heart; not a wizard in sight.

What we have to live with will follow
us forever, like the cases that carry
our writing workshops—the cases,
not us yet, on wheels. We are sharing
the borders of our limited lives. She is,

*"Trying to figure out who I am, now
that I'm not the person I was."* I am
thinking Frost was lucky. He had a choice
of roads in his yellow wood. I have miles
to go, a book to write, pain to share.

The road I see is a long allee, only fog
at the end, and I go alone, deciding who
this I, this me, is, as I go. But Alice and me
have shared this climb; we'll find the way
to the next level.
That is when the Little Voice, you know, the one
that speaks on the wind, tells the truth,
ready or not, to me and my bear (my silent
brown-eyed Zen master). It reminds me what
Tennyson's aging Ulysses, sitting on his rock,
knew, "Though much is taken, much abides."

Then the Little Voice turns the tables,
quoting at me a small poem of my own:
When you wake and thank the universe for
all your blessings, listen for 'You're welcome'
in the sunrise, in your granddaughter's eyes."

CODA

I am more at peace.
I know what I know.
My body has been teaching
my soul who I really am.
The course is not over yet.

BIBLIOGRAPHY
And a list of books which have been helpful to me on my journey

American Heart Association Complete Guide to Women's Heart Health: The Go Red for Women Way to Well-Being and Vitality. New York: Clarkson/Potter Publishers, 2009.

Bernard, Christian, MD. *Fifty Ways to a Healthy Heart.* London: Thorsons, 2001.

Chilnick, Lawrence. *Heart Disease: An Essential guide for the Newly Diagnosed.* Philadelphia, Pennsylvania: DaCapo Press, 2008.

Chodron, Thubten. *How to Free Your Mind: Tara the Liberator.* Ithaca, New York: Snow Lion Publications, 2005.

Cohen, Jay S. MD. *What You Must Know About Statin Drugs and Their Natural Alternatives.* Garden City Park, NY: Square One Publishers, 2005.

Cousins, Norman. *The Healing Heart: Antidotes to Panic and Helplessness.* New York: W.W. Norton, 1983.

Dellmore, Doug and the editors of Prevention Magazine. *Pain-Free Living.* Emmaus, PA: Rodale Press, 2000.
————————————*New Choices in Natural Healing.* Emmaus, PA: Rodale Press, 1995.

Devi, Nischala Joy. *The Healing Path of Yoga: Alleviate Stress, Open Your Heart and Enrich Your Life.* Cincinnati, OH: Three Rivers Press, 2000.

Efteriades, ,John A.MD and Teresa Coulin-Glaser MD. *The Woman's Heart: An Owner's Manual.* Amherst, NY: Prometheus Books,2008.

Gottlieb, Bill, and the editors of Prevention Magazine. *New Choices in Natural Healing.* Emmaus, PA: Rodale Press, 1995

Guarneri, Mimi, MD. *The Heart Speaks: A Cardiologist Reveals the Secret Language of Healing.* New York: Touchstone Books, 2006.
————————————-*The Science of Natural Healing.* Chantilly Virginia: The Great courses, 2012.

Guiness, Alma, editor. *Family Guide to Natural Medicine: How to Stay Healthy in the Natural Way.* Pleasantville, NY: The Reader's Digest Association, Inc., 1993.

Houston, Mark C., MD, MS. *What Your Doctor May Not Tell You about Heart Disease.* New York: Grand Central Publishing, 2012.

Huddleston, Peggy, RN. *Prepare for Surgery, Heal Faster: A Guide to Mind/Body Techniques.* Angel River Press, 2012.

Isaacs, Nora. "The Cutting Edge of Trauma Treatment: Healing Through the Body" Kripalu Center for Yoga and Health, (Summer, 2009. Cited with permission.)

Judith, Anodea. *Eastern Body, Western Mind: Psychology and the Chakra System as a Path to the Self.* Berkeley/Toronto: Celestial Arts, 1996.

Kabat-Zinn, Jon. *Coming to Our Senses: Healing Ourselves and the World Through Mindfulness.* New York: Hyperion, 2005.

Kastan, Kathy. *From the Heart: A Woman's Guide to Living Well with Heart Disease.* Cambridge, MA: Da Capo Press, 2007.

Miles, Pamela. *Reiki: A Comprehensive Guide.* New York: Jeremy Tarcher/Penguin, 2006.

Moyers, Bill. *Healing and the Mind. New York: Doubleday, 1998.*

Myss, Caroline, PhD. *Anatomy of the Spirit: The Seven Stages of Power and Healing.* New York: three Rivers Press,1996.

Naprastek, Belleruth. *Staying Well with Imagery.* New York: Wellness Central, 1995.

————————————————————*Invisible Heroes: Survivors of Trauma and How they Heal.* New York: Bantam Books, 2004.

Oz, Mehmet, MD. *Healing From the Heart: How Unconventional Wisdom Unleashes the Power of Modern Medicine. New York: Plume/Penguin, 1998.*

Pert, Candace. *Molecules of Emotion: The Science Behind Mind-Body Medicine.* New York: Scribner, 1997.

Piscatella, Joseph C. *Positive Mind, Healthy Heart: Take charge of Your Cardiac Health One Day at a Time.* New York: Workman Publishing Company, Inc, 2010.

Piscatella, Joseph C.and Barry A. Franklin, MD. *109 Things You Can Do to Prevent, Halt and Reverse Heart Disease.* New York; Workman Publishing Company, Inc., 2011.

Quest, Penelope. *Self-Healing with Reiki.* New York: Jeremy Tarcher/Penguin,2012.

Rankin, Lissa MD. *Mind Over Medicine: Scientific Proof that You Can Heal Yourself.* Carlsbad, CA: Hay House Inc, 2013.

Roizen, Michael, MD and Mehmet C. Oz, MD. *YOU Staying Young: the Owner's Manual for Extending Your Warranty.* New York: Simon & Schuster/Free Press, 2007.

Sinatra, Steven MD and James C. Roberts MD with Martin Zucker. *Reverse Heart Disease Now: Stop Deadly Cardiovascular Plaque before It's Too Late.* New York: John Wiley & Sons, 2005.

Songs of Tara: Devotional Music to the Goddess of Liberation Liner Notes. Boulder, Colorado: Sounds True, 2011.

Steinbaum, Suzanne, DO, with Eve Adamson. *Dr. Suzanne Steinbaum's Heart Book: Every Woman's Guide to a Heart-Healthy Life.* New York: Avery/Penguin Group, USA: 2013

Vanderhaeghe, Lorna, MS, with Michelle Hancock and Byron Collyer. *A Smart Woman's Guide to Heart Health.* Markham, Ontario, Canada: Fitzhenry and Whiteside, 2010.

Weil, Andrew MD. *Healthy Aging: A Life-Long Guide to Your Well Being.* New York: Anchor Books, 2005.

Wilber, Ken. *Integral Psychology.* Boston: Shambala Press, 2000.

Williamson, Craig. *Muscular Re-training for Pain Free Living.* Boston: Trumpeter Books, 2007.

RESOURCES

BOOKS:

At the start, we recommend two books which have too many listings to have them included separately here:

Gottlieb, Bill, and the editors of Prevention Magazine. *New Choices in Natural Healing.* Emmaus, PA: Rodale Press, 1995.

The Resource section contains 16 pages of associations with a list of books for each specialty.

Dellmore, Doug, and the editors of Prevention Magazine. *Seniors Guide to Pain Free Living.* Emmaus, PA: Rodale Press, 2000.

Features excellent safety guides for the use of essential oils, vitamins and herbs.

ASSOCIATIONS

This list is by no means complete. It has been compiled by noting those resources which are repeatedly recommended in various books, and in some cases, my own experience with them. By exploring these various sites, you will find that each one opens up a whole new world of information and ideas. You may find that different sources give different points of view, but you will have a chance to evaluate these in terms of your own needs and make your own decisions about your health. At the very least, they will help you to know what questions to raise with your doctors and other health care practitioners

The American Heart Association, National Center
7272 Greenville Avenue
Dallas, TX 75231
800-242-8721
http://www.americanheart.org
Their website offers extensive sections of information on all aspects of heart health.

The Mended Hearts, Inc. (affiliated with the AHA)
http://www.mendedhearts.org
Can refer you to a support group in your area.

Academy for Guided Imagery
10780 Santa Monica Blvd.
Los Angeles, CA 90025
800-726-2070
www.healthy.net/agi

Academy of Integrative Health and Medicine
5313 Colorado Street
Duluth, MN USA
218-525-5651
info@aihm.org

American Academy of Medical Acupuncture
1970 East Grand Avenue, Suite 330
El Segundo, CA 90245
310-364-0193
www.medicalacupuncture.org
A professional organization for physician acupuncturists

American Association for Music Therapy
PO Box 80012
Valley Forge, PA 19484
610-265-4006
A certification organization

American Association for Oriental Medicine
4101 Lake Boone Trail, Suite 201
Raleigh, NC 27607
919-787-5181
www.aaom.org/aahome.htm
A professional association for nonphysician acupuncturists.

American Association for Applied and Therapeutic Humor
342 North Main Street , Suite 301
West Hartford, CT 06117
888-747-2284
e-mail: info@aath.org
Offers information, membership, conferences, humor resources and publications.

American Board of Physician Specialties
5550 West Executive Drive
Tampa, FL 33609
813-433-2277
http://www.abps.org
Represents 24 medical specialty boards and establishes high standards for medical certification. Use it to make sure that your specialist is truly certified in his/her medical specialty.

American Board of Integrative and Holistic Medicine
5550 West Executive Drive
Suite 400
Tampa, FLA 33609
813-433-2277
www.ABOIM.org
Information on certification, conferences, a directory of Integrative Medicine specialists from all over the country.

American Chiropractic Association
11701 Clarendon Blvd.
Arlington, VA 22209
703-276-2593
www.amerchiro.org/aca

American Music Therapy Association
8455 Colesville Road, Suite 1000
Silver Spring, MD 20910
301-589-3300
www.musictherapy.org

The Heart Truth:
A National Awareness Campaign on Women and Heart Disease
http://www.hearttruth.gov
You may order a Red Dress pin

American Massage Therapy Association
820 Davis Street, Suite 100
Evanston, Il 60201-4444
847-864-0123
www.amtamassage.org
Offers referrals to qualified therapists

Center for Mindfulness in Medicine, Healthcare and Society
University of Massachusetts Medical Center
Stress Reduction Clinic
55 Lake Avenue North
Worcester, MA 016555
508-856-2656
www.umassmed.edu/cfm/
Jon Kabat-Zinn, PH.D., is the founder and director of this clinic using mindfulness-based stress reduction

Complementary Care Center
Columbia Presbyterian Medical Center
Milstein Hospital Building
177 Fort Washington Avenue
New York, NY 10032
www.nyp.org/services/complimentary.html
Drs. Memet Oz and Jerry Whitworth, Directors

Guarneri Integrative Health at Pacific Pearl
6919 LaJolla Boulevard
LaJolla, CA 92037
858-459-6919
www.pacificpearllajolla.com
State-of-the-art Western medicine meets the best of global healing traditions. Mind, body, and spirit are treated as one.

healthy.net
A health resource center–a virtual health village where you can access products,
information and services to help you create wellness

Heart Sisters
A Canadian site all about women and heart disease from the perspective of Carolyn Thomas, a Mayo Clinic-trained heart attack survivor, speaker, blogger and advocate for women's health.
Independent and self-funded
www.myheartsisters.org

Himalayan International Institute of Yoga, Science and Philosophy
RR 1 Box 400
Honesdale, PA 18431
800-822-4547
www.himalayaninsti
Teaching classical yoga for modern-day life

International Association of Yoga Therapists
PO Box 251563Little Rock, AR 722259 28-541-0004
www.iayt.org/

International Institute of Reflexology
P.O. Box 12642
St. Petersburg, FL 33733
813-343-4811
e-mail: info@reflexology-usa.net

Mind/Body Medical Institute
Division of Behavioral Medicine
New England Deaconess Hospital
185 Pilgrim Road
Boston. MA 02215
617-632-9530

National Institutes of Health (NIH)
National Center for Complementary and Alternative Medicine (NCCAM)
900 Rockville Pike
Office of Alternative Medicine
Bldg. 31, Room 5-B-38
Bethesda, MD208992
800-531-1794

Preventive Medicine Research Institute
900 Bridgeway, Suite 2
Sausalito, CA94965
415-332-2525, ext. 222

Reflexology Research
P.O. Box 35820
Albuquerque, NM 87176
800-624-8773

Reiki Alliance
PO Box 41
Cataldo, ID 83810

Scripps Center for Integrative Medicine
10820 North Torrey Pines Road
LaJolla, Ca 92037
858-554-3300
Offers comprehensive integrated care. A well-respected center.

UCSF HealtheHeart Study
555 Mission Baay Blvd, South
Suite 161, SanFrancisco, CA14158
This is a national mobile health initiative
>HealtheHeartStudy<coordinator@healtheheartstudy.org<

WebMD
http://www.webmd.com
A respected source of information about many medical conditions, including heart disease

WomenHeart:
The National Coalition for Women with Heart Disease
818 18th Street, NW
Suite 930
Washington, DC
202-728-7199
http://www.womenheart.org
Information on locations of over 600 support groups across the country, and how you can start one in your area. The website offers much in the way of both information and support for heart patients.

CD'S AND AUDIO TAPES:
For music suggestions, please see the chapter on music. A number of artists are listed there.

Health Journeys Audio Tapes
891 Mol Drive
Suite C
Akron, OH 44310
800-800-8661
Offers evidence-based guidance for help with stress, illness, medical procedures, emotional resilience, wellness and behavioral change, featuring leading practitioners and teachers in the mind-body health field.

NOTES

[1] Steinbaum, *Suzanne Steinbaum's Heart Book*, 30

[2] Women's Heart, An owner's Manual, 52

[3] Ibid, 14

[4] Ibid, 36

[5] Rimmerman, *Cleveland Clinic Guide to Heart Attacks, 66*

[6] Ibid, 36

[7] Ibid, 68

[8] Chilnick, *Heart Disease: An Essential Guide for the Newly Diagnosed,* 160

[9] Cousins, *The Healing Heart: Antidotes to Panic and Helplessness, 107*

[10] Cohen, *What You Must Know About Statin Drugs & Their Natural Alternatives,* 42

[11] Isaacs, "The Cutting Edge of Trauma Treatment: Healing Through the Body," 57

[12] Fiore, *New Choices in Natural Healing,* 114

[13] Naparstek, *Everyday Heroes: Survivors of Trauma and How They Heal,* 108

[14] Ibid, 106

[15] Ibid, 77

[16] Oz, *YOU Staying Young,* 78

[17] Naparstek, *Everyday Heroes: Survivors of Trauma and How They Heal,* 87

[18] Ibid, 135

[19] Ibid, 32

[20] Moyers, *Healing and the Mind,* 326

[21] Moyers, *Healing and the Mind,* 326

[22] Ibid, 324

[23] Ibid, 335

[24] Cousins, *The Healing Heart,* 26

[25] Devi, *The Healing Path of Yoga,* 5

[26] Myss, *Anatomy of the Spirit: The Seven Stages of Power and Healing,* 47-48

[27] Oz, *YOU Staying Young,* 79

[28] Judith, *Eastern Body, Western Mind,* 1x

[29] Ibid, 4

[30] Oz, *Healing from the Heart,* 113-114

[31] Myss, *Anatomy of the Spirit,* 68

[32] Pert, *Molecules of Emotion,* 35

[33] Ibid, 34

[34] Moyers, *Healing the Mind,* 188

[35] Ibid, 186

[36] Oz, *YOU Staying Young,* 114

[37] Judith, *Eastern Body, Western Mind: Psychology and the Chakra System as a Path to the Self,* 18

[38] *Readers Digest Family Guide to Natural Medicine,* 88

[39] Chilnick, *Heart Disease: The Essential Guide for the Newly Diagnosed,* 287-288

[40] Cousins, *The Healing Heart: Antidotes to Panic and Helplessness,* 140

[41] Oz, *From the Heart: How Unconventional Wisdom Unleashes the Power of Modern Medicine,* xv

[42] Naperstek, *Invisible Heroes: Survivors of Trauma and How They Heal,* 149

[43] Naparstek, *Staying Healthy With Guided Imagery,* 360

[44] Guarneri, *The Heart Speaks,* 47

[45] Sinatra and Roberts, *Reverse Heart Disease Now: Stop Deadly Cardiovascular Plaque before It's Too Late,* 224

[46] Oz, *YOU Staying Young,* 186

[47] Ibid, 187

[48] Steinbaum, *Suzanne Steinbaum's Heart Book,* 284-285

[49] Kaplan, *The Seniors Guide to Pain-Free Living,* 73

[50] Ibid, 75

[51] Oz, *YOU: Staying Young,* 45

[52] Ibid, 102

[53] Gottlieb, *Prevention Magazine.* 115

[54] Gottlieb, Bill, and the editors of Prevention Magazine, *New Choices in Natural Healing,* 29

[55] Kastan, *From the Heart,* 95

[56] Weil, *Healthy Aging,* 269

[57] Dunbar, *AARP Magazine,* Feb/Mar 2012, 15

[58] Sinatra, *Reverse Heart Disease Now: Stop Deadly Cardiovascular Plaque before It's Too Late,* 190

[59] Kastan, *From the Heart: A Woman's Guide to Living Well with Heart Disease,* 90

[60] Spiegel, *Seniors Guide to Pain-Free Living,* 98

[61] Efteriades and Coulin-Glaser, *The Woman's Heart-an Owner's Manual,* 139

[62] Ibid, 101

[63] Guarneri, *The Heart Speaks,* 82

[64] Steinbaum, *Heart Book,* 236-238

[65] Spiegel, *The Senior's Guide to Pain-Free Living,* 126

[66] Ibid, 126-127

[67] Oz, *Healing from the Heart,* 89-99

[68] Ibid, 90

[69] Halpern, *New Choices in Natural Healing,* 124-125

[70] Ibid, 125

[71] Ibid, 126-127

[72] Kastan, *From the Heart: A Woman's Guide to Living with Heart Disease,* 93

[73] Halpern, *New Choices in Natural Healing,* 132

[74] Neparstek, *Staying Well with Guided Imagery,* 198

[75] Naparstek, *Everyday Heroes, Survivors of Trauma and How They Heal,* 149-150

[76] Ibid, 360

[77] Quest, *Self-Healing with Reiki ,* 15

[78] Myss, *Anatomy of the Spirit,* 36

[79] Pert, *Molecules of Emotion*, 275
[80] Ibid, 243
[81] Oz, *YOU, Staying Young,* 315
[82] Borysenko, *New Choices in Natural Healing,* 119
[83] Moyer, *Healing and the Mind*, 116
[84] Ibid, 134
[85] Naparstek, *Invisible Heroes,* 322

SOME HELPFUL CHECKLISTS

Notice that these are questions, NOT directions. Sometimes, writing things down can be a great help in clarifying where you are in becoming a responsible partner in your own healing. I am not a medical authority, just a survivor.

> ➤ Do you know your blood pressure? Record it here

_____

> ➤ Body Mass Index and Weight?

_____

> ➤ Cholesterol levels? Total _____
> HDL _____LDL _____

> ➤ How much sleep do you usually get

_____

> ➤ Do you smoke? _____

> ➤ If you have prescriptions from your doctor, do you take them as you should? _____

> ➤ If you take OTC meds, does your doctor know about all of them?

_____

> ➤ Do you get regular exercise?

_____

> How much and in what form?

_____

> Can you list the general symptoms of a heart attack?

_____

> Can you list the unusual symptoms of a woman having a heart attack?

_____

_____

> If these symptoms appear in you or in others, how long should you wait to call 911? _____
The American Heart Association now says five minutes.

> Should you drive or wait for an ambulance? _____
Hospitals and the AHA say DO NOT DRIVE.

IF YOU ARE PRE-SURGERY

Once again these are questions NOT directions. I am not a medical authority, just a survivor.

> ➤ Have you asked all the questions you need to ask about the procedure?

> ➤ Have you had someone with you to take notes in case you forget what was said?

> ➤ Have you informed your surgeon about ALL the meds you take, both RX and OTC?

> ➤ Do you know that some meds may have to be stopped?

> ➤ Have you assembled a support group–family, friends, etc, for when you come home? (Do not be shy about asking for help.)

> ➤ What have you done to calm yourself? Music, counselor, prayer, massage–whatever works for you?

> ➤ Have you asked about music during surgery? Some hospitals allow it, but you may need to ask.

> ➤ Will you observe the prep directions exactly? (Be sure to ask if you do not understand any of them.)

A CHECKLIST FOR HEALING

And one more time. These are questions, NOT directions because I am not a medical authority, just a survivor.

> ➤ Do you have all the proper phone numbers to contact your doctor or hospital?

> ➤ Have you made sure to understand all your instructions before leaving the hospital?

> ➤ Are you following those instructions carefully?

> ➤ Are you taking all meds exactly as directed?

> ➤ Are you doing your exercises, no matter how boring?

> ➤ Are you laughing every day

> ➤ Are you reporting any problems to your doctor?

> ➤ Will you sign up for your twelve weeks of a hospital cardiac program? Medicare will pay.

> ➤ Have you planned to do regular exercise after your twelve week program?

> ➤ Do you have plans to keep actively mentally?

> ➤ As you move on with your recovery, are you willing to keep an open mind about some forms of healing that you have not tried yet?

ABOUT THE AUTHOR

Marylou Kelly Streznewski holds a Master's degree in English from the College of New Jersey. Her career has included theater, journalism and teaching writing from high school through college and community levels. Streznewski is an eclectic writer, publishing in poetry, fiction and non-fiction.

Two chapbooks, *Rag Time* and *Woman Words* (J.G. Whitthorne Press) are housed in the chapbook collection at Poet's House in New York. A third chapbook, *Dying with Robert Mitchum* was released by Aldrich Press in 2015. Short fiction has appeared in *The St. Anthony Messenger, The Bucks County Writer, The New England Writer's Network, The U.S.# 1 (Princeton NJ) Sumer Fiction Issue, Best New Writing of 2015,* where it was a finalist for the Gover Prize, the Amazon Shorts program on Amazon.com, and is featured in *Genesis,* a new literary quarterly.

In non-fiction, Streznewski is the author of *Gifted Grownups: The Mixed Blessing of Extraordinary Potential* (John Wiley & Sons), a study of one hundred gifted adults. It has been translated into Chinese and published in Taiwan, is used as a textbook in graduate courses, and appears in over one hundred libraries worldwide.

Streznewski lives on an acre in Bucks County Pennsylvania with her husband Tom, where she is working on her first novel.

For more information visit: http://streznewskiwrites.com

DISCUSSION QUESTIONS

1. Were there any items on the "Helpful Checklists" that you did not know about?
2. Why did you feel the need to read this book?
3. How close is your experience to that of the author?
4. What surprised you?
5. Did the poetry help you to understand Streznewski's experience?
6. Will you be more energetic in speaking up to doctors as a result of reading this book?
7. Studies show that trauma can impair the language function of the brain, which explains why some people say, "I don't want to talk about it," after a bad experience. What has been your experience—does talking help or not?
8. Were any of the healing modalities completely new to you? Which ones might you be likely to try?
9. Have you experienced any of these modalities and did they work for you?
10. How important do you think support is from the following:
    a. Family
    b. Medical personnel
    c. Those who have "been there"
    d. Reading books like this
    e. Medications
11. How would you describe what you have learned from reading this book?

Feedback about these questions is welcome!

Please include number of people, ages, and location of your group to Marylou Streznewski: strez7@verizon.net

Made in the USA
Middletown, DE
05 February 2017